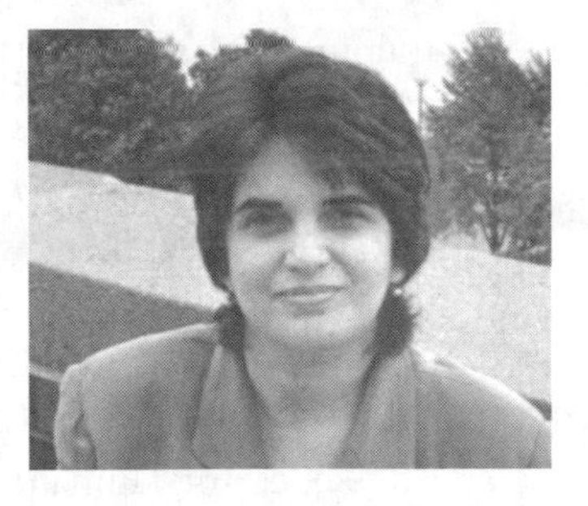

Nina M. Silverstein, PhD, is Associate Professor and Director of the Undergraduate Gerontology Program, University of Massachusetts Boston Gerontology Institute and Center, ... ty Service.

Dr. Sil... tion for he... f Alzheimer ... decade, she has worked closely with the Alzheimer's Association on projects relating to the Association's Helpline, its Safe Return Program, respite care, support groups for family caregivers, and home safety adaptations for people with dementia. She recently completed a term as chairperson of Board of Directors of the Association's Massachusetts Chapter, and now serves on its Advisory Board. She also serves on the Board of Directors of the Council on Aging in Needham, Massachusetts.

A graduate of the Heller School, Brandeis University, Dr. Silverstein has been publishing and presenting on aging issues at major national conferences since the outset of her career over 20 years ago. Among other affiliations, she is a Fellow of the Gerontological Society of America, and an active member of the Association of Gerontology in Higher Education. Recent articles have appeared in the *Journal of Gerontology and Geriatric Education* and the *Journal of Women and Aging*. Dr. Silverstein resides in Needham, Massachusetts with her husband Irwin and has two daughters in college, Ilana and Julie.

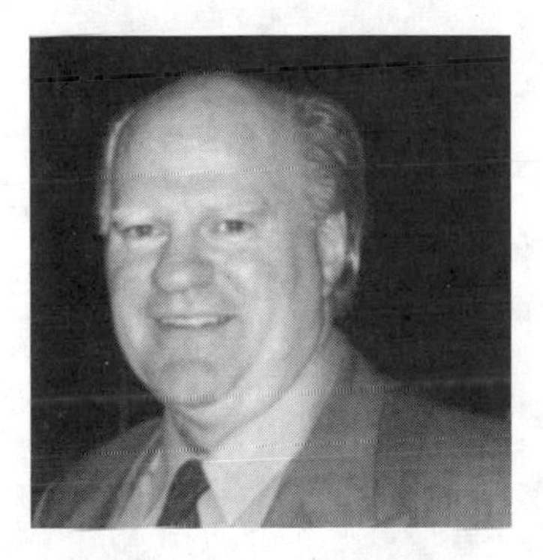

Gerald Flaherty has been with the Massachusetts Chapter of the Alzheimer's Association since 1989. As Director of Special Projects, he coordinates the national Safe Return Program in Massachusetts, the chapter's Medical & Scientific Advisory Committee, and its media relations. In his previous work as an analyst in the Massachusetts state Senate, he helped draft legislation to assist caregivers of people with dementia. His mother died of Alzheimer's disease.

Safe Return is a registry-based program which coordinates efforts to locate and recover people with dementia who become lost. It is operated 24 hours a day by the Alzheimer's Association with support from the U.S. Justice Department. In his role as Safe Return Coordinator, Mr. Flaherty has been involved in some 800 lost patient cases, and has provided training to police, firefighters, EMS, search and rescue personnel, and elder care workers throughout Massachusetts. He has helped to develop training materials and videos for the Safe Return Program, and serves on several local and national advisory groups. His articles have appeared in the *American Journal of Alzheimer's Disease and Related Disorders*, the *Journal of Elder Abuse & Neglect*, and the *Attorney General's Law Enforcement Newsletter*. Mr. Flaherty lives in southeastern Massachusetts with his wife, Diane, and their family.

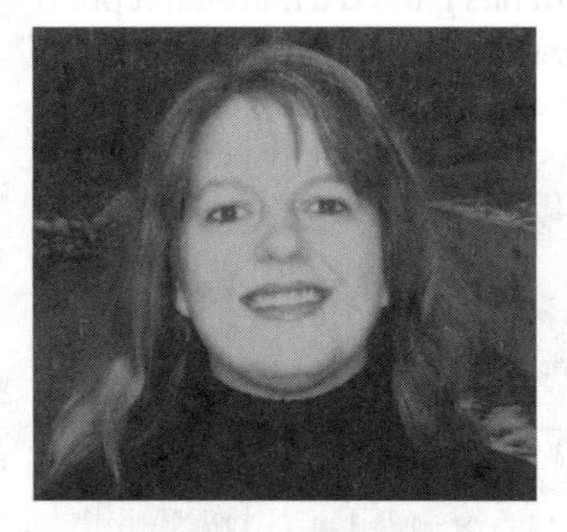

Terri Salmons Tobin, PhD, is Associate Director of Research at Advocates for Human Potential, Inc., in Sudbury, MA. She received her PhD in Gerontology from the University of Massachusetts Boston in 1999. With a dissertation titled, *Wandering, Getting Lost, and Alzheimer's Disease: Influences on Precautions Taken and Levels of Supervision Provided by Caregivers*, Dr. Tobin's work on this book was also influenced by her position as an Alzheimer's respite caregiver and "walking buddy" during graduate school. Her current areas of research include those involving caregiver issues, Alzheimer's disease and wandering behavior, housing and serious mental illnesses, and co-occurring disorders. Dr. Tobin currently resides in Southborough, MA with her husband, James, and her newborn daughter, Ashleigh.

Dementia and Wandering Behavior

Concern for the Lost Elder

Nina M. Silverstein, PhD
Gerald Flaherty
Terri Salmons Tobin, PhD

SPRINGER PUBLISHING COMPANY

Springer Publishing Company, Inc.
536 Broadway
New York, NY 10012-3955

Acquisitions Editor: Helvi Gold
Production Editor: Sara Yoo
Cover design by Susan Hauley

02 03 04 05 06 / 5 4 3 2 1

Library of Congress Cataloging-in-Publication Data

Dementia and wandering behavior: concern for the lost elder / Nina M. Silverstein, Gerald Flaherty, Terri Salmons Tobin, authors.

p. cm.

Includes bibliographical references and index.

ISBN 0-8261-4262-1

1. Dementia. 2. Dementia—Complications. 3. Mental illness—Treatment. 4. Psychology, Pathological. I. Silverstein, Nina M. II. Flaherty, Gerald. III. Tobin, Terri Salmons. IV. Title.

RC521 .S56 2002
616.8'3—dc21

2001057664
CIP

Printed in the United States of America by Capital City Press.

This book is dedicated to all those whose personal and professional commitment promotes dignity and safety for people with Alzheimer's disease and other dementing illnesses.

Contents

Part III: Creating a Safe Environment

Foreword

Alzheimer's is rapidly becoming the epidemic of the 21st century. Today an estimated 4 million Americans suffer from this devastating illness. And unless we find a cure, this number is expected to explode to 14 million by 2050 as the Baby Boomers come of age.

In 1999, along with my good friend Chris Smith (R-NJ), I established the bipartisan Congressional Task Force on Alzheimer's Disease to enlist our colleagues in the battle against this epidemic. One hundred and fifty-eight members strong, the Task Force has played a key role in the increase of funding for Alzheimer's research by over $100 million since its inception. This investment in science is crucial to finding a cure, and I have no doubt that one day children will have to look to the history books to learn about Alzheimer's disease. But until that day arrives millions of Americans will continue to face the challenges of Alzheimer's not only as patients, but also as family caregivers living with an immense responsibility.

Until we find a cure, this nation must continue to create and to invest in programs designed to improve the lives of those affected by this illness. One crucial and unique federal program is called Safe Return. The Safe Return Program was established nationwide to assist in the identification and timely recovery of people with Alzheimer's and related dementias who wander and become lost. Each year, the Alzheimer's Task Force has been successful in securing full funding for this incredibly important program.

Unless one has dealt directly with an Alzheimer's patient, it's difficult to imagine the day-to-day challenges associated with caring for a loved one with the disease. The stress is further amplified by the need to keep constant and vigilant watch over the ambulatory Alzheimer's patient as the disease progresses. Public awareness of Alzheimer's disease is crucial for a variety of reasons—but it is perhaps most crucial in order to provide a community safety net for the Alzheimer's patient who is lost and wandering

In *Dementia and Wandering Behavior: Concern for the Lost Elder,* authors Nina Silverstein, Gerald Flaherty and Terri Salmons Tobin provide an excellent resource for building public awareness. This easy-to-read book offers concrete suggestions for the range of professional caregivers in community and institutional settings, for people with dementia and their families in the community, as well as for first-responders such as police and search and rescue personnel.

Dementia and Wandering Behavior: Concern for the Lost Elder speaks to the risks associated with wandering behavior and demonstrates that acknowledgment of these risks leads to early precautions to avoid them. This in turn can lead to reduced stress on caregivers, greater autonomy for people in the earlier stages of the disease, and increased safety for anyone with Alzheimer's who is ambulatory. Ultimately, *Dementia and Wandering Behavior: Concern for the Lost Elder* provides invaluable information to help Alzheimer's patients remain longer and more secure with their friends and families in the community, and more safe with their caregivers in facilities. The authors embrace the goal that we as a nation should all embrace—the goal of enhancing the quality of the lives of people with dementing illnesses like Alzheimer's disease.

REP. EDWARD J. MARKEY, CO-CHAIR
Congressional Task Force
on Alzheimer's Disease

Preface

Dementia robs the afflicted of their daily experiences and future prospects. It robs us all of their companionship and wisdom. The great burden of dementia is not from the patient's forgetting his neighbor's name, it's from wandering into his neighbor's home. Our first obligation is to protect the patient and this book provides practical advice for achieving that goal.

Alzheimer's disease creates deficits in a variety of domains. It is not simply the loss of memory, but also of language, judgment, and spatial orientation. The mode of presentation and sequence of progression is highly idiosyncratic, but one-third to one-half of the patients have spatial orientation loss early in their illness and these patients are thought to be especially prone to wandering.

Our work at the University of Rochester, and that of our colleagues around the globe, is revealing the neural mechanisms of spatial disorientation in dementia. Alzheimer's patients who get lost in familiar surroundings have an impaired capacity to see the patterned visual motion of optic flow. Optic flow informs us about the speed and direction of our self-movement and about the three-dimensional structure of the visual environment. Alzheimer's patients do not get lost because they have forgotten where they are going, rather, they get lost because they cannot keep track of where they have been.

After facing the tragedy of a dementia diagnosis, these patients confront a succession of painful realizations: realizing that the lifelong habit of automobile driving must be abandoned, that routine independent excursions must be curtailed, and that an independent household can no longer be maintained. Episodes of wandering and getting lost accelerate the relentless cycle of isolation and loss of independence.

Health care professionals, caregivers, and family members struggle to keep patients safe and help them adjust. Unfortunately, appropriate responses are commonly impeded by a failure to fully recognize current impairments and further changes on the horizon. The best way to prevent this is by understanding the disease and its consequences. That understanding can begin with this book.

This book is divided into three parts. The first part deals with defining dementia as the progressive loss of functional capacity due to neurological deficits. A review of the pertinent literature is provided that emphasizes the enormity of the problem of wandering, and its devastating consequences. The diverse manifestations of dementia, its epidemiology, and its differential diagnosis are then described. This presentation offers a framework that is helpful to the professional while providing level of detail that is suitable for those who are new to the subject.

The second part deals with community responses to wandering. The presentation of general principles is extensively illustrated by specific examples from the authors experience and the literature. The focus on wandering allows a comprehensive description of the problem and a detailed elaboration of what various community programs and institutions can do to help. In particular, the utility of the Safe Return Program is aptly exemplified and important resources for advice and useful appliances are provided.

The third part of the book addresses the needs of a variety of individual care providers. Chapter 7, on creating a safe home environment, provides the benefits of extensive experience in a clear presentation. This chapter, and others, include a number of useful lists that concisely describe the dos and don'ts of home care. Chapters 8 and 9 describe what is needed to create a supportive living program that educates staff and protects patients. Finally, Chapter 10 provides expert advice for the many community-based professionals, from social services to law enforcement, who are often called upon to rescue the wandering elder.

Alzheimer's disease impairs sensory processing, robbing patients of the ability to extract experience from sensation. This undermines their capacity to share in everyday life and isolates them in a world of their own. This is the world in which they wander. Until dementia can be controlled, cured, and prevented we must make every effort to bridge these worlds with compassion and knowledge. I commend the authors on this worthwhile contribution to that effort.

CHARLES J. DUFFY, MD, PHD
Department of Neurology
University of Rochester Medical Center,
Rochester, New York

Acknowledgments

We hope this book can be of some help to those who each day face the challenge of finding their way through the ordinary routines of their lives. For finding our own way to the book, and through it, we acknowledge the several million people who have Alzheimer's disease or a related disorder, and the hundreds working in the Alzheimer's Association's Safe Return Program nationwide.

Many others helped. Our list is not prioritized, and we suspect we may have missed a few. We thank the caregivers who participated in both our quantitative and qualitative research efforts. In the interim between the Silverstein and Salmons study in 1996 and the Salmons study in 1999, author Salmons (now Salmons Tobin) was a "walking buddy" for the late Clayton Sibley. Insights gained through her experiences with Clayton and his wife Diane contributed greatly to her doctoral research and to the awareness we hope to generate by using parts of it here.

The Gerontology Institute and Center at the University of Massachusetts Boston supported author Silverstein's initial exploration into this topic by providing resources under the auspices of the Elder Action-Research class of the Gerontology certificate program. UMass provided a supportive environment for Salmons Tobin, who received a graduate award while there from the Association of Gerontology in Higher Education and the AARP Andrus Foundation to support her doctoral research on wandering behavior.

We thank the staff and volunteers at the Massachusetts Chapter of the Alzheimer's Association; Joanne Koenig-Coste, Elaine Silverio, and the members of their respective early stage patient support groups who shared their fears and concerns about wandering and becoming lost; the family of the late Charles Mayers; Paul Raia; Brian Johnson; Curt Rudge; Robert

Koester; Jim Zagami; Jeanette Rosa-Brady; John Scheft; Ed Markey; and Charles Duffy.

And a special thanks to Irwin, Ilana, and Julie Silverstein, and Edward and Surrie Melnick; Jed and Ashleigh Tobin; Diane Lopes Flaherty and the late Lillian Flaherty.

Part I

Introduction

Most of the time I forgot I had Alzheimer's in the earliest days until I realized one morning that I could not visually map out in my mind where I was supposed to go that day and it was a place I frequented. I had a hard time coming to grips with this loss of visual memory. It was this realization that made me talk to my family and get help. I have not worried about getting lost because, since that day, I do not leave the house by myself . . . never. To not be able to create a map in your mind is so scary.

Member of a support group for people with early stage dementia
Summer 2001

Introduction

For people with Alzheimer's disease or a related dementia, wandering away from home or a care facility and becoming lost is the most life-threatening behavior associated with their illness. For family and professional caregivers, it can be the most emotionally wrenching event in their caregiving experience. And while "forgetfulness" may be the symptom which most often leads families and elder care professionals to seek a diagnosis for a loved one or client, it is the frightening experience of a wandering incident that just as often leads them to seek other helpful services (Silverstein & Salmons, 1996).

Public awareness concerning Alzheimer's disease has increased in the past decade, but for the estimated 4 million people in the United States with Alzheimer's or a related dementia, these services remain few and far between. Although 70 to 80% of Americans with dementia live in the community (Crosby, et al., 1993; Hall, et al., 1995), nationally less than 2% receive any supportive assistance such as homemaking, home health care, or day care (Alzheimer's Association, 1990). The most likely reasons for the low level of supportive assistance appear to be that at-risk elders do not self report their medical or other problems, and public resources to locate high-risk elderly or to serve people with Alzheimer's disease and their caregivers are uniformly lacking (Raschko, 1991; Silverstein, 1984).

At least 20% of people with dementia who live in the community are living alone, with estimates reaching 44% in some geographic regions (U.S. Congress, 1990). They are our neighbors and, for those in the elder service field, our clients. And they are, by definition, at risk. People with serious memory problems who live alone and have no services are at continuous imminent risk of wandering and becoming lost (Flaherty & Raia, 1994). Their often isolated environment lends itself to the psychiatric complications of dementia, such as hallucinations and delusions, which, in turn, are conducive to wandering. As Flaherty and Raia wrote, "If the best current, practical and humane treatment for people with dementia is the almost constant reassurance they receive from others, then people with dementia who live alone spend their lives in an unenviable place, where the real fears associated with our noisy and sometimes dangerous cities, or our isolated suburbs, are only enhanced by the effects of dementia" (p. 84).

This population constitutes what social researcher Raymond Raschko (1991) has called "a social policy time bomb." One behavior, in particular, has alerted elder care professionals to the ticking of this time bomb—the increasingly well-documented propensity of people with dementia to wander away from home and become lost. This behavior places them at risk whether they live alone or with involved caregivers. Wandering has been cited as a major cause of hospital admission (Sanford, 1975), of serious physical risk (Silverstein & Salmons, 1996) and of death (Koester & Stooksbury, 1994).

Wandering has also been described by in-home caregivers as the least manageable (Young, 1988) and most-mentioned (Calkins & Namazi, 1991) problem they face. It is a primary factor leading to placement in a long-term care facility (Ferris, 1987). In the early and middle stages of the disease, the behavior is manifest. The Alzheimer's Association (1998) estimates that as many as seven out of ten people with Alzheimer's disease or a related dementia will wander from home or a care facility and become lost during the course of the disease. Many will do so repeatedly (Silverstein & Salmons, 1996). In reviewing data from law enforcement and other agencies, one search and rescue expert (Koester, 2001) estimates that more than 127,000 critical wandering incidents involving people with dementia occur each year, of which only about 34,000 are reported to police. Rowe and Glover (2001) found that less than 4% of memory-impaired adults who wander away from home are able to return unassisted, and that "individuals who have regularly taken independent walks in the community on a regular basis may, on any given day, become lost and find themselves unable to return home on their own" (p. 13).

For all involved, a wandering episode is an emotionally wrenching experience. Wandering is not just another problem associated with dementia—no caregiver, for example, will call the police for problems with incontinence. Wandering is a major hallmark of dementing illness, and as such it cannot be ignored.

The purpose of this book is to enable readers to recognize wandering behavior when it occurs, to enable them to understand that wandering is indeed a life-threatening behavior, and to respond to the oft heard comment,

"There's nothing we can do about it." And we include people with Alzheimer's disease and related disorders among our readers. Particularly for people with early stage Alzheimer's, knowledge about ways to deal with the risk of wandering and becoming lost addresses issues of autonomy, not just safety. As more people are diagnosed earlier in the disease process, autonomy and self-determination will almost certainly become larger issues for patient and caregiver alike. This is why we have looked at ways, from the Alzheimer's Association's Safe Return Program to emerging, high-tech personal locator technologies, which can help people with dementing illnesses remain safe and relatively independent for as long as possible.

The book is also intended to promote the largely unexplored notion that this behavior is not simply an isolated symptom of Alzheimer's disease and other dementias, but part of a process that culminates in someone with a dementing illness becoming lost. This process involves multiple interacting factors, including biochemical changes in the brain, lifelong patterns of coping with stress, and environmental stimuli (Alzheimer's Association, 1993). For example, our "cognitive mapping" skill is associated with the parietal lobe of the brain, which controls spatial orientation. This skill enables us to get from point A to point B and back without getting lost. The parietal, temporal and occipital lobes connect in the posterior region of the brain, and comprise the brain's visual cortex. In studying impairment of the visual cortex in Alzheimer's, Duffy, Tetewsky, and O'Brien (2000) identified a phenomenon they termed "motion blindness," or the lack of motion perception. They found that people with Alzheimer's disease experienced an impaired ability to process optic flow—that complex flow of information the eyes send to the brain as we move through our environment. People with Alzheimer's experienced increasing difficulty determining if it is they—or the objects around them—that are moving. This offers one explanation for the disorientation that can lead a person with Alzheimer's wandering and becoming lost, even quite early in the disease process. In fact, Rosa-Brady and Dunne (1999), in an article about visual problems in Alzheimer's disease, report that several of the participating elders in the Duffy study who had no apparent memory loss nevertheless tested abnormally for motion blindness, and later developed probable Alzheimer's disease. According to Rosa-Brady and Dunne, this leads Duffy to believe that "motion blindness may precede memory problems in some people with Alzheimer's. Since motion blindness was an early indicator for Alzheimer's in some test subjects, Duffy hopes his findings will become useful in diagnostic testing, and feels they may also be helpful in identifying people with Alzheimer's who are at increased risk for wandering."

But while wandering behavior has been associated with damage to the visual cortex early on in the disease process, people with dementia who become lost may also be experiencing fear, seeking exercise or companionship, looking for a childhood home, trying to get to a former place of employment, or be driven by a number of other desires or impulses. Additionally, the home or care facility from which they disappeared may or may not constitute an emotionally secure or physically safe environment. All of these factors and more come into play when someone wanders and becomes lost. Viewed in this context, this difficult behavior can often be managed.

A full exploration of how wandering behavior relates to various occupational category within the dementia care field follows in the chapters of Part II, and in Part III we will offer specific suggestions on interventions and responses for specific professions—from community and long-term care providers to police and search and rescue personnel. In Part II we will also discuss wandering from home, from a day or long-term care facility, whether by foot, by car, or by other means. Information will be categorized in such a way as to make it easily accessible for the sometimes different but always related purposes of the various professions. We hope to make this a practical, efficient, expedient resource, a sort of quick-reference book on wandering behavior for professionals across the elder care field. Part I, on the other hand, consists largely of the kinds of background information we thought necessary to illuminate the core problem of wandering and becoming lost. This information may also be useful to researchers, faculty, and students in age-related disciplines. In chapter 1, for example, the literature review provides a broad but easy to digest overview of Alzheimer's disease and the related dementias. Such a general look at dementia will aid in our understanding of one of the most common behaviors associated with it. In chapter 2, following a full review of the research literature, we will come to a working definition of wandering behavior. Chapter 3 profiles the dementia wanderer, and offers insights drawn not only from the work of researchers, but from the immediacy of the experiences of family caregivers. In Part II, chapter 4 details some current community responses to wandering behavior, with a special focus on the Alzheimer's Association's national Safe Return program.

Our literature review in chapter 2 produced some useful definitions which fit particular research parameters for particular studies. Further research will no doubt focus in other ways on other aspects of the behavior. Our purpose in revisiting these definitions was not so much to formulate a working definition of our own as it was to clarify precisely what it is about wandering behavior that in our opinion *most* warrants the attention of elder care professionals.

Whatever the cause, wandering requires immediate intervention. The National Institute of Nursing Research (1994) identified wandering as a top-priority area of study. We certainly agree. Elder care providers need to address the wandering process before it creates the kinds of crises which an overburdened elder service system is not currently equipped to resolve in the safest, wisest or most humane way. Our own studies, together with our reading of the literature and direct experience in cases involving people with dementia who have wandered and become lost, have led us to the following three assumptions. They are the impetus behind this book, and guide us throughout.

- If someone with a dementia can walk, that person can wander and become missing.
- If someone with a dementia is missing, that person is lost.
- And if someone with a dementia is lost, that person is at risk of harm.

CHAPTER 1

Alzheimer's Disease and Related Dementias: An Overview

Alzheimer's is a progressive, degenerative disease which attacks the brain and results in impaired memory, thinking, language and behavior. It is the most common cause of dementia. Dementia itself is not a specific disease, but a group of symptoms which may accompany certain diseases or physical conditions (Alzheimer's Association, 1990). In Alzheimer's, the symptoms of dementia include a decline in intellectual functioning so severe that people with the disease gradually lose the ability to take care of themselves without assistance. There are a number of other dementing illnesses which produce similar symptoms and the same endpoint as Alzheimer's disease. These are referred to as the Alzheimer-related dementias, and are the focus of the section *Causes of Alzheimer's Disease*, which follows. There is currently no lasting medical treatment and no cure for progressive, dementing illnesses such as Alzheimer's disease.

The disease was first described by Dr. Alois Alzheimer in 1906, although it has been with us for centuries. It is also seen in the literature as Alzheimer's Dementia, Senile Dementia of the Alzheimer's Type (SDAT), or simply AD. It is sometimes, incorrectly, called "senility." Senility, however, is not a disease. We all experience some physical and mental changes as we age. Older people, for example, typically experience some musculoskeletal problems and some hearing and vision loss. They also may experience minor cognitive changes for which they can easily compensate. These changes are a part of normal aging.

The progressive cognitive decline triggered by Alzheimer's disease is not part of the normal processes we associate with aging. The brain's billions of neurons, or nerve cells, communicate by using chemicals. In Alzheimer's disease, nerve cells in areas of the brain responsible for memory and other thought processes degenerate for reasons which are under intense investigation by research scientists. Some of the nerve cells most damaged by the disease communicate by using a chemical called acetylcholine, which helps transmit electrical nerve impulses important to memory. The brains of people with Alzheimer's appear to lose the ability to make acetylcholine, or to maintain acetylcholine levels in amounts necessary for normal cognitive functioning. Early in the disease process, Alzheimer's affects nerve cells in the hippocampus, the brain's memory center. It also disrupts the passage of electrochemical signals between nerve cells in the cerebral cortex, the brain's outer layer. Gradually, it causes the death of cells in areas throughout the brain which control memory, perception, judgment, motor skills, and other abilities. As one person with the disease put it, "It's as if I hear things and they get into the wrong slots, which make no sense to me at all" (Davis, 1989).

Another significantly affected area of the brain is the visual cortex which, as mentioned in the *Introduction,* influences our ability simply to get from one place to another, and back, without getting lost. The disease also causes disorientation and frequent difficulty relating to the environment (Roberts & Algase, 1988). This damage can and usually does lead to wandering behavior.

Alzheimer's disease is generally defined as falling into two categories.

1. Late-onset, or sporadic, Alzheimer's occurs in people who are typically over age 65 and represents upwards of 90% of cases.
2. Early-onset, or familial, Alzheimer's occurs in approximately 1 to 9% of cases. Familial Alzheimer's appears to have a definite genetic link and tends to affect people who are younger, typically in their 40s, 50s, or early 60s.

Signs of the Disease

The Alzheimer's Association has identified ten warning signs of progressive memory loss. (See *Stages of the Disease*, below, for more on manifestations of the disease.)

- Recent memory loss which affects job, or other, skills. (We have all misplaced our keys or forgotten a telephone number. People with Alzheimer's disease, however, may forget how *to use* the keys or the phone. And because of the *short term memory loss* typical of the

disease, they will become increasingly unable to absorb or retain new information.)
- Difficulty performing familiar tasks. (Cooking or serving a meal, for example.)
- Problems with language. (People with dementia forget simple words or substitute an inappropriate word for the forgotten one. A faucet may become a "water dripper," for example. They will often repeat themselves, asking the same question many times.)
- Disorientation as to time and place. (They may forget appointments or get lost on their own street.)
- Poor, or decreased, judgment. (They may step out into heavy traffic against the lights, for example, or leave the house in a snowstorm dressed only in pajamas.)
- Problems with abstract thinking. (Alzheimer's disease affects our ability to think logically, or to perform math. The numbers in the checkbook in time become meaningless.)
- Misplacing things. (And sometimes putting them in inappropriate places.)
- Changes in mood or behavior. (Going from calm to tears to anger for no apparent reason.)
- Changes in personality. (Including profound confusion, suspicion, or fear.)
- Loss of initiative. (Someone with dementia may require cues and prompting to become involved in a familiar activity.)

Alzheimer's disease is by far the most common cause of these symptoms of dementing illness.

Causes of Alzheimer's Disease

The genetics of Alzheimer's disease are more complex than those of most other diseases, in part because there are multiple ways in which the disease develops. There is also a need to clarify the role, if any, of nongenetic factors, although there is little compelling evidence for an infectious origin for Alzheimer's, or for a toxic-environmental origin such as aluminum (Selkoe, 1993). Many factors contribute to the cause and progression of Alzheimer's, and there are multiple genes involved. So far, 4 genes have been very clearly associated with the disease, although others are currently under investigation. Three of the 4—presenilin 1 (PS1) on chromosome 14, presenilin 2 (PS2) on chromosome 1, and the amyloid precursor protein (APP) on chromosome 21—are identified with early-onset, familial Alzheimer's disease.

For the far more common late-onset, sporadic Alzheimer's, two genes have been identified. One of them, apolipoprotein E (APOE), was found on chromosome 19 and comes in three forms, or alleles, known as e2, e3, and e4. Every person has two alleles, one from each parent. Current thought is that the 4 to 8% of people with one or two e4 alleles are at higher risk for late-onset Alzheimer's disease (Roses, 1995). The e4 allele on the APOE gene appears to increase the level of amyloid beta protein in the brain. Amyloid beta protein deposits, called plaques, form in the brains of people with Alzheimer's disease. These plaques are thought to cause the brain's nerve cells to become inflamed and die (although there is still some debate over whether the plaques are the cause or the result of cell death). Other research indicates that the APOE gene may have a stronger influence on the age of onset of Alzheimer's disease, than on the risk of getting the disease (Breitner, et al., 1999).

Studies have also found that low education is a risk factor for Alzheimer's. While this does not mean that people with PhDs do not get the disease, one study of nuns living in a Milwaukee convent found that low linguistic ability—determined from essays written when the nuns were in their twenties—predicted eventual development of the disease (Snowdon, et al., 1996). This study was seen as one more indication that Alzheimer's disease may begin long before people show clinical symptoms. In fact, whatever the cause, the disease process may begin well before symptoms appear, by some estimates 20 or more years before clinical diagnosis (Snowdon, et al., 1996; Reiman, et al., 1996).

Despite the obvious complexity of Alzheimer genetics, there is compelling reason for optimism about the discovery of a cause and cure. We have learned more about Alzheimer's disease in the last 5 years than we did in the previous 30.

Other Causes of Dementia

There are several other dementing illnesses which are both progressive and irreversible (Alzheimer's Association, 1997). After Alzheimer's, the most common degenerative memory disorder is vascular dementia. This type of dementia produces the same endpoint as Alzheimer's disease but by a different process. On autopsy, it is not uncommon to find evidence of both Alzheimer's disease and vascular dementia in the same person.

Multi-infarct dementia is one of the most common vascular dementias. It is caused by multiple small strokes, or infarcts, within the brain. Infarcts are caused when a branch of a blood vessel becomes clogged by small clots, or emboli, from the heart or neck arteries. The blockage deprives an area of brain tissue of oxygen and nutrients. The symptoms of multi-infarct dementia depend on which specific area of the brain has been deprived, and consequently damaged. Strokes in the parietal lobe, which controls spatial orientation, can cause people with multi-infarct dementia to wander and become lost. This behavior and other symptoms are similar to those in Alzheimer's disease. Unlike Alzheimer's, however, in which there is a slow but steady progression of symptoms, multi-infarct dementia often progresses in a step-like fashion, with symptoms "plateauing" until further infarcts cause further cognitive decline.

Pick's disease (and related frontal-temporal lobe dementia) was once confused with Alzheimer's, as the symptoms are similar. People with Pick's disease, however, show a more dramatic atrophy of the frontal and temporal lobes of the brain. The disease usually begins between the age of 40 and 60. Disturbances in personality and behavior among people with Pick's disease may precede, and be more severe than, their memory problems.

Binswanger's disease is another type of vascular dementia, in which stroke-like changes occur in the white matter deep within the center of the brain. It is closely associated with hypertension.

Parkinson's disease affects more than 1 million Americans (Alzheimer's Association, 1999). It can often be treated successfully with drugs. Symptoms include a loss of control of muscle activity resulting in tremors, stiffness, and speech impediments. In the late stage, usually 10 years or more into the disease, Parkinson's can result in a dementia similar to Alzheimer's disease. But because the physical problems in Parkinson's are so overwhelming, the early signs of dementia are often missed. A person with Parkinson's dementia may lose the physical ability to button a shirt, for example, long before losing the cognitive ability necessary to perform that task. For someone with Alzheimer's, the reverse may be true.

Lewy body disease is a relatively recently observed disorder of the brain. Its symptoms can appear as a combination of Alzheimer's and Parkinson's, with both cognitive impairment and abnormal physical movements.

Although the cause of brain degeneration may be different in the different types of dementia, people with these diseases seem to share cognitive and behavioral problems which put them at risk of wandering and becoming lost.

Other causes of dementia are considerably less common, and their rates of progression vary greatly. What they have in common, however, is they are progressive, degenerative, and can produce the same confusion and disorientation which lead people with Alzheimer's disease to wander and become lost.

Huntington's disease is a hereditary disorder which causes intellectual decline and psychiatric problems, as well as involuntary movements of the limbs or facial muscles. Huntington's can be positively diagnosed. Its progression cannot be stopped, but its physical and psychiatric symptoms can be controlled with drugs.

Creutzfeldt-Jakob disease is another rare and fatal brain disease which causes memory problems and affects muscular coordination. It is caused by a transmissible agent called a "prion," and progresses very rapidly.

Normal pressure hydrocephalus is yet another rare disease, caused by a blockage in the flow of cerebrospinal fluid, causing a buildup of fluid on the brain. Symptoms include difficulty in walking, memory loss, and incontinence. It can sometimes be corrected with surgery, by the insertion of a shunt to divert the fluid away from the brain.

An additional and sometimes overlooked population at risk of wandering behavior includes people with mental retardation, among whom the incidence rate for Alzheimer's disease is nearly twice that of the general population (Lai, 1992). For people with Down syndrome, which is the most common cause of mental retardation, Alzheimer's disease is a virtual certainty. Research indicates that there may be a link between trisomy 21 (being born with an extra, or third, copy of all or part of chromosome 21), which causes Down syndrome, and a small percentage of cases of familial Alzheimer's thought to be influenced by the APP gene on chromosome 21. On autopsy, brain tissue from people with Down syndrome shows patterns of plaques and tangles as well as chemical deficits similar to those seen in brains affected by Alzheimer's disease. Because memory loss may be more difficult to detect in people with mental retardation—when there's no clear baseline for short-term memory, for example—the first symptoms noticed are more likely to be personality or behavioral changes, such as wandering (Antonangeli, 1996).

There are also a number of conditions listed below which can mimic the symptoms of Alzheimer's disease. Nutritional deficiencies and depression are noteworthy, because both can result from the neglect and social isolation too often experienced by elders, as is polypharmacy, because it describes the situation of so many elders who are prescribed a number of different medications which can cause a dangerous reaction when taken simultaneously. More germane to this book, however, is alcoholism, principally because alcoholics are disproportionately represented among homeless populations, particularly in our cities. As the homeless alcoholic ages, his continued drinking damages brain cells and affects his orientation to time and place. As his ability to sustain himself on the street diminishes, he comes to the attention of the law enforcement, medical, and social work systems, often because he is lost and confused.

The treatable illnesses which impair memory are known as pseudodementias. They include: depression, alcoholism, drug reactions, thyroid disorders, nutritional deficiencies, brain tumors, and infections such as AIDS, meningitis, and syphilis (Alzheimer's Association, 1997).

Prevalence Rates

There are an estimated 4 million people in the United States who suffer from Alzheimer's disease or a related neurological disorder (Evans, et al., 1990), although an analysis of 18 different prevalence studies in the U.S. and Europe found the number to be closer to 2.1 million people (U.S. General Accounting Office, 1998). Prevalence rates are greater for women than for men, which may be due to the longer life expectancy of women. Alzheimer's disease is the fourth leading cause of death among adults, after heart disease, cancer, and stroke (Katzman, 1976).

Over 90% of Americans with Alzheimer's are age 65 or older (Alzheimer's Association, 1993). One frequently cited study of prevalence rates, which assessed more than 3,600 people living in the community, found that among all those age 65 and older, 10.3% had probable Alzheimer's. The highest rate in that study, 47.2%, occurred in those over age 85 (Evans, et al., 1989).

But while prevalence estimates in the many studies vary, there is unanimity on two points:

1. prevalence rates increase sharply with age, doubling about every 5 years up to age 85; and
2. most people with the disease are in the 75–89 age group.

These findings take on added significance in light of 1990 and 2000 U.S. Census data placing the 80+ age group among the fastest growing segments of the general population.

Diagnosis

From 12 to 19% of suspected Alzheimer's cases prove, after a neurological evaluation using the clinical diagnostic criteria for Alzheimer's disease, to be some other medical condition (Tierney, et al., 1988). Since some of these other conditions—such as the alcoholism, depression, and other conditions mentioned above—are treatable and even reversible when diagnosed in a timely fashion, elder care professionals are strongly advised to pursue full diagnostic evaluations for all those experiencing memory loss, confusion, and disorientation. Accurate diagnosis is also important for other reasons. Without it, useful therapies and medications which can sometimes delay the symptoms of dementia may inadvertently be withheld. Additionally, family and professional caregivers need to know the name and nature of the disease they are dealing with before they can begin to address problem behaviors such as wandering. And just as important, people with the disease who are still able to participate in decisions about their future deserve that opportunity. In the early stage of the disease, they generally seem to be aware of their memory problems. Many people with Alzheimer's also seem to do better after they have been told of their diagnosis. Raia (1994) speculates that this may be because they realize that they do not have an emotional illness and that their memory problems are due to a brain disease that is beyond their control. Supporting that view, a family caregiver whose husband was diagnosed with dementia wrote, "*Organic* (emphasis hers), physical, not psychosomatic, not within the control of the patient. This word was a source of enormous relief to us" (Kunkemueller, 1998).

There is no single test to diagnose Alzheimer's disease. A definitive diagnosis is only possible with a brain autopsy or, in rare cases, with a brain biopsy. The brain tissue of someone with Alzheimer's disease is distinguished from those affected by other types of dementia by the presence of tangles of fibers, called neurofibrillary tangles, and clusters of degenerative nerve endings, called neuritic plaques, which appear in areas important for memory and intellectual functioning. As mentioned in the section *Causes of Alzheimer's Disease*, these plaques are thought to cause the death of brain cells, which are not replaced. The Alzheimer's brain literally shrinks, its weight ultimately diminished by 30 to 40%. People with the disease may lose a third of their brain mass (Roses, 1995). Another characteristic of Alzheimer's is the reduced production of certain brain chemicals, especially acetylcholine and somatostatin, which are necessary for normal communication between nerve cells.

The highly accurate differential diagnosis is the suggested method of testing for dementia (Small, Rabins, et al., 1997), and consists of a detailed medical history, physical exam, neuroimaging techniques such as a CT scan or MRI, and neuropsychological testing. Neuropsychological testing often consists of having the memory-impaired person perform some combination of the following: name the day, month, and year; remember three key words stated at the beginning of the exam; count backwards by seven; draw a clock with the minute and hour hands at a specified time. The more comprehensive differential diagnosis is performed by a team of clinicians, ideally with caregiver input, with the object of ruling out any other possible causes of symptoms. Some of the specialist roles outlined below are interchangeable.

TABLE 1.1 Diagnostic Specialist Table

SPECIALIST	ROLE
Neurologist	Does neurological testing (EEG, CT scan, or MRI)
	Assesses for seizures
Neuropsychologist	Tests memory, language, reasoning, arithmetic skills
Psychiatrist	Takes medical and social history
	Assesses for clinical depression
	Evaluates overall test results
	Manages all medications
Internist/Geriatrician/ Family Practitioner	Does complete physical examination
	Acts as primary care physician
Nurse/Social Worker	Refers to community supports
	Advises on behavioral management

Genetic Testing

Having a gene associated with Alzheimer's does not mean a person will develop the disease. Having the APOE-e4 gene is a risk factor, for example, but not a predictive factor. And since there is no cure for Alzheimer's, the value of genetic testing for all but a minute number of people with a clear genetic predisposition to familial Alzheimer's disease is questionable. Even then, the rare person knowing he or she has a causative gene may experience unnecessary anxiety, anger, depression, and stress. And although various legislation has been introduced to address genetic discrimination, such discrimination by insurers, or employers, remains a possibility. The Alzheimer's Association strongly recommends that anyone planning a genetic test also undergo pre and posttest counseling. This advice should be taken into consideration by anyone considering genetic testing for any dementing illness.

Life Expectancy

Average life expectancy from the appearance of symptoms—not from point of diagnosis or point of contact with the elder service system—is just over

8 years (U.S. Congress, 1987), with symptoms usually occurring 2–4 years before diagnosis (Berg & Morris, 1994). As mentioned under *Causes of Alzheimer's Disease*, however, the slow disease process may begin decades before clinical symptoms actually appear. Although 8 years is the average life expectancy from the appearance of these symptoms, people with Alzheimer's can sometimes live for 20 years or more from that point. Caring for them all too frequently depletes families of their physical, emotional, social, and financial resources.

Stages of the Disease

Alzheimer's disease progresses in three loosely defined stages. People with the disease gradually lose their orientation as to time, place, and person, roughly in that order. Damage to particular skills related to time, place, and person may overlap, however, because many functions, including memory, occur in widely dispersed areas of the brain. Our emphasis in this book is on the early and mid stages of the disease, delineated below, when people with dementia are more mobile and thus more apt to wander and become lost.

Early stage

Early on, people are often aware of their illness and require less supervision. With support, they carry on with minimal changes in lifestyle. This is not to say that they do not wander and become lost in this early stage of the disease. They do. The difference at this early point is that they still have the cognitive ability to ask for help, to recall where they live, or even, depending on the stress of the moment, to recall a phone number. The usual early-stage duration is 1 to 3 years. Areas of decline include:

- Short-term memory
- New learning
- Language (especially word-finding problems)
- Planning and calculation
- Behavior (e.g., impulse or temper control, lowered inhibitions)
- Personality (e.g., flattened affect, frustration, less drive)
- Cognitive mapping (i.e., getting from point A to point B and back without getting lost)
- Fine motor control and reaction time
- Work productivity

- Doing complex tasks and understanding directions
- Depression

Middle stage

In the broad middle stage of the disease, people are unable to perform everyday tasks without supervision. They have poor memory of the recent past but may still remember more distant events. There is increased disorientation to time, in particular, and also to place and person. The usual duration is 2–8 years. Additional areas of decline include:

- Judgment
- Decision-making
- Expressing and understanding language, word repetition
- Expressing emotions appropriately
- Recognizing familiar people
- Personal safety (e.g., getting lost)
- Independence related to activities of daily living (the ADLs—e.g., bathing, dressing, toileting, grooming, eating)
- Psychiatric health (e.g., anxiety, paranoia, hallucinations, and the catastrophic reactions, or super anxiety attacks mentioned below under *Psychiatric issues*)

Late stage

In the late stage of the disease, people are usually unable to communicate, have poor recent and remote memory, are apathetic, and require complete care. The usual duration is 1–3 years. Final areas of decline include:

- Mechanics of chewing and swallowing
- Major organs controlled by the autonomic nervous system

While still physically active and able to communicate, as in the early or mid stages of the disease, people with Alzheimer's can nevertheless have difficulty with the critical analysis involved in making simple judgments and decisions (Moss & Albert, 1988). People moderately impaired with Alzheimer's can also have great difficulty with routine activities of daily living, such as preparing and eating their food, paying bills, and maintaining personal hygiene. As mentioned, these difficulties extend to such simple tasks as finding the way from one familiar point to another. As the person's cognitive mapping skills progressively and inevitably diminish, wandering, in particular, becomes a life-threatening behavior.

The following case not only provides an example of that particular difficulty, but also illustrates just how deceiving appearances can be when we attempt to gauge risk in Alzheimer's disease.

> Mr. E. took the same one-mile walk each day, which involved negotiating a busy intersection near his home in the city. He was reported to state Elder Protective Services by police after becoming lost on three occasions, and the Protective Services caseworker asked that Alzheimer's Association representatives sit in on a family conference. Otherwise quite caring, the family refused to recognize the risks associated with these walks. Nor was the Protective Services worker altogether convinced of the degree of risk when Mr. E.'s son, after accompanying his father on one such walk, reported that his father went directly to the crosswalk at the intersection and waited for the WALK signal before stepping off the curb.
>
> That behavior not only seemed to demonstrate his father's awareness of the fast moving cars and trucks in the street, but convinced the son that his father still had the intellectual capacity to avoid the potential danger they posed. Since habit and analysis (of visual information, in this instance) are two different things, our interpretation of Mr. E.'s actions was very different. By going to the crosswalk, Mr. E. was reacting to his less compromised long-term memory. And by waiting for the pedestrian light before stepping into the street, he was reacting to cues from his son, who had remained at his father's side on the curb until the appropriate signal flashed.
>
> We suggested the son once more accompany his father on the same walk, but this time stay a short distance behind his father and not alert him to his presence. Once again, the son reported that his father went directly to the crosswalk, looked up at the traffic signal—which read DO NOT WALK—and did indeed look both ways at the heavy traffic before stepping right into it. The son was close enough to draw him back safely. He returned home as convinced as we were that pure luck alone had been keeping his father alive (Flaherty & Raia, 1996).

Excess Disability

Excess disability is a common term associated with Alzheimer's disease and describes the loss of capacity by someone with the disease to perform a specific task—dressing herself, for example—before that capacity is likely to be lost, given the stage of the disease. It has been defined as having more cognitive impairment than can be explained by the disease itself. According to the Alzheimer's Association (1993), "Causes of excess disability can include intercurrent illnesses, pain, medications, or poor hearing/vision." While some of the following conditions may correspond to what could reasonably be expected at a given stage of Alzheimer's disease, others may not. For someone with the disease who wanders and becomes lost, these various disabilities, whether "excess" or not, have both medical and psychiatric implications which considerably elevate the risk of harm.

Medical issues

There are more burn injuries to the elderly than to all others in the United States except those under age two, and the risk of such injuries is compounded by dementia (Petro, et al., 1989). Mental status, as well, significantly increases the risk of injury from falls among the elderly (Morse, et al., 1987). As for general physical health, people with dementia have been shown on average to have more than three coexisting medical conditions (U.S. Congress, 1990), including, among other problems: hearing impairment, cardiac illness, arthritis, and hypertension (Figure 1.1). Older people in general are more susceptible than others to hypothermia and dehydration. The added medical problems of older people with Alzheimer's disease who wander from home or a facility and become lost only magnify their physical vulnerability.

Psychiatric issues

A study of 217 mild to moderately impaired people with Alzheimer's disease, all of whom were living in the community, found that they experienced

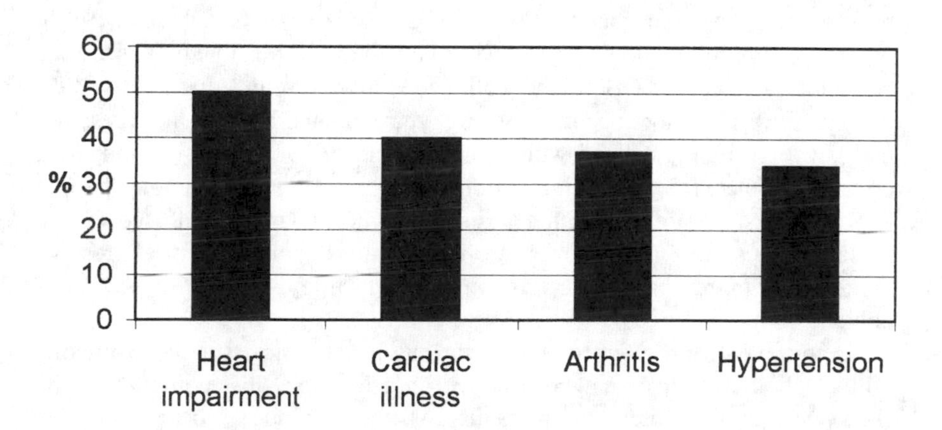

FIGURE 1.1 Coexisting medical conditions.

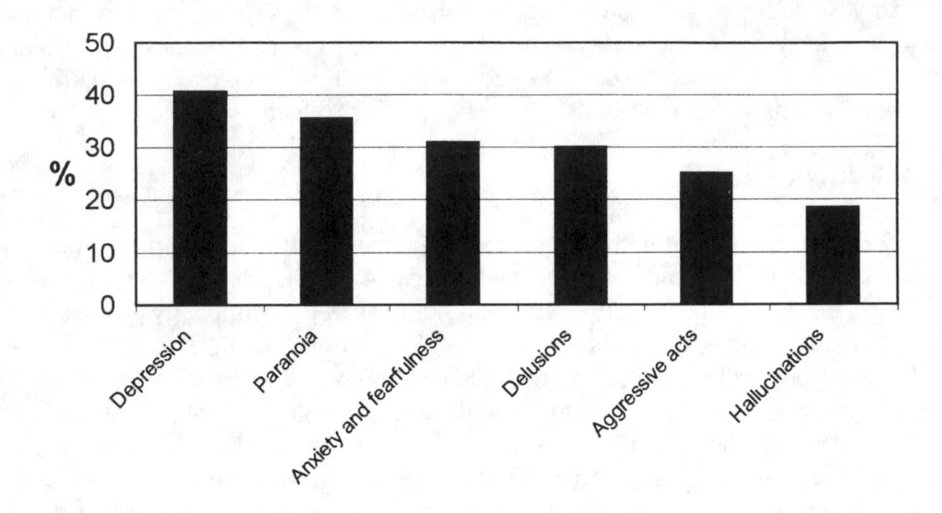

FIGURE 1.2 Psychiatric complications.
From Mendez, et al., 1990.

the following psychiatric complications: depression, paranoia, anxiety and fearfulness, delusions, aggressive acts, and hallucinations (Figure 1.2) (Mendez, et al., 1990).

Another study followed 32 recently diagnosed people with Alzheimer's for 6 years, all of them living in the community, and found that symptoms of psychosis only worsened as the disease progressed (Rosen & Zubenko, 1991).

Before continuing, however, we would add a clarifying note on aggressive behavior. A study by Gilley and colleagues (1997) found that nearly 80% of aggressive behaviors occurred during a care-related activity like dressing, bathing, or toileting, all of which involve close, even intrusive, physical contact. Further, the aggressive actions were more common among people in the later stages of Alzheimer's disease, who are more confused. Since these people require more care, there is a greater opportunity for aggressive or, to use a more appropriate term in light of Gilley's findings, "reactive" behavior.

In any event, the effect of these various psychiatric issues on someone with Alzheimer's disease who wanders and becomes lost compounds the risks posed by the more obvious medical issues. Any one of these issues can completely obviate whatever ability that person might have had to find his or her own way home, or even to ask for help. Additionally, a behavioral phenomenon called *catastrophic reaction* is not uncommon among people with Alzheimer's under stressful conditions. This is a sort of super anxiety attack, usually lasting 15–20 minutes. It usually involves crying and pacing, but can include agitated behavior such as throwing things or knocking things over. Of special note here, a catastrophic reaction can also include running away from a caregiver. Worse yet, in a number of cases (see *Chapter 10*) where a wanderer has been missing for several hours or more, it includes getting into dense brush and other generally inaccessible and overlooked places, with disastrous results.

Family caregiving issues

The well caregiver is not immune to a type of excess disability, in that the typical family caregiver is a woman in her 70s who has three chronic medical problems of her own to deal with in addition to her spouse's dementia (Alzheimer's Association, 1990).

A caregiver whose husband's body was found less than a quarter of a mile from their home following a wandering incident typifies many of these problems. "I'm 79 years old and I have a heart condition," she told an Alzheimer's Association representative. "I just couldn't chase after him."

Caregiving takes an obvious toll. In addition to the attendant medical problems, providing care for someone with dementia has long been recognized as a cause of stress, a circumstance aptly caught in the title of one of the best-selling books for caregivers, *The 36-Hour Day*. The lengthy experience often leads to depression in family caregivers. Some studies have reported that nearly 50% meet the diagnostic criteria for depression (Raia, 1994). Sleep disturbance was cited by 70% of family caregivers as a reason for nursing home placement (Pollak & Perlick, 1987). The effects of their experience on caregivers' preexisting medical conditions is palpable. In one study (Chenoweth & Spencer, 1986), about 21% of family caregivers institutionalized relatives because the caregivers themselves became ill or injured. Most of those caregivers were spouses in their 60s or 70s.

Specific interventions will be discussed in future chapters, but it should be said here that family support groups provide a helpful forum for caregivers to share feelings, concerns, and information, and to assist one another in coping with the psychological effects of caring for someone with dementia.

Driving issues

We mention driving in this section only because the automobile represents an instrument of potentially instant disability, excess or otherwise. We will discuss Alzheimer's wanderers who become lost while they are driving in a later chapter. But for the moment, a brief review of some of the literature on driving and Alzheimer's may be helpful. While the research regarding the driving skills of people mildly impaired with Alzheimer's disease may not offer hard and fast recommendations, no researcher debates the need for regular retesting and constant vigilance of even the most mildly impaired patients who drive (Kapust & Weintraub, 1992; Hunt, et al., 1988). A study conducted at Johns Hopkins University found that over 40% of people with early Alzheimer's who drove had been in an accident after their diagnosis and that 44% routinely got lost (Lucas-Blaustein, et al., 1988). Furthermore, researchers who examined the brains on autopsy of elderly people who died in car crashes found that one-third showed clear evidence of early stage Alzheimer's disease (Johanson, et al., 1997).

But, as the following case indicates, relinquishing the car keys may be problematic:

> Mr. J., with a 2-year-old diagnosis of Alzheimer's disease, dependent on cognitive cueing by his wife to dress himself but insistent on driving his car, claimed that he would most certainly know when he should stop driving. "When I've had an accident," he said. Incredibly, both his family and his caseworker were comfortable with this line of reasoning (Flaherty & Raia, 1994).

What was needed in this case (literally an accident waiting to happen) was a real-life demonstration, through the state's Department of Motor Vehicles or other appropriate testing center, of Mr. J.'s capacity to drive safely.

Here are some things to consider in assessing when someone with Alzheimer's needs to stop driving: Alzheimer's disease affects reaction time and visual-spatial relationships; wanderer cases take much longer to resolve when the lost person is driving; and the risk is not only to the person with Alzheimer's but to the public. Additionally, the American Psychiatric Association has recommended that doctors write prescriptions directing people with Alzheimer's not to drive, based on evidence that they are more likely to cause crashes, even in the earliest stages of the disease (*Associated Press*, 1997).

People demonstrate many different capacities in their daily lives—they bathe and dress themselves, plan and cook meals, make financial decisions, give advice to their children. For someone with Alzheimer's disease, however, the competence to perform in these "capacities" can exist at different levels at different times. Typically, people with Alzheimer's lose their awareness of their deficits, and if they are aware, will minimize them. There is another distinction to keep in mind when assessing the risks faced by people with Alzheimer's disease: "No" may mean something else, such as "I don't understand," or "I'm afraid." It is important to learn to respond not only to the words, but to the emotions behind them.

Treatments

There is accelerating activity in several treatment areas, often in cooperation with the Alzheimer research centers funded by the National Institutes for Health, and with funding of research by the Alzheimer's Association.

Currently 4 drugs are approved by the U.S. Food and Drug Administration specifically for Alzheimer's. They are available only by prescription. Their costs are covered by some health insurers. They act by inhibiting the enzyme acetylcholinesterase, thereby slowing the breakdown of acetylcholine in the brain. Increasing the amount of acetylcholine in the brain allows nerve cells to communicate better and thus improves memory. Unfortunately, none of these drugs prevents cell death, and once the disease progresses to a stage when there is little acetylcholine left in the brain, they lose their effectiveness.

Treatment of dementia caused by vascular disease and stroke, such as multi-infarct dementia and Binswanger's disease, also involves the treatment of underlying conditions such as heart disease, high blood pressure, diabetes, smoking, or high cholesterol levels. Treating these risk factors can sometimes slow the progression of these types of dementia.

While there are many other pharmacological and, potentially, genetic treatments in development, it is a better understanding of the psychology of dementia—how a person thinks, feels, communicates, compensates, and responds to change, to emotion, to love—which may bring some of the biggest breakthroughs in treatment. An entire therapeutic model, called Habilitation Therapy, has been built on the premise that the last brain function to fail in people with dementia is the ability to feel and express emotion (Raia & Koenig-Coste, 1996).

In fact, according to a report on current treatments by Lombardo (1997) in the newsletter of the Alzheimer's Association's Massachusetts Chapter, it was a psychoeducational intervention targeting family caregivers in the home which has had the biggest impact to date on how long people with dementia stay alive, functional, and living at home. In a study of 206 people with dementia and their caregivers, the caregivers received initial, intensive individual and family counseling, with continuously available follow-up counseling and support groups. After 8 months, these caregivers were less likely to be depressed than caregivers in the control group, a benefit which not only persisted after completion of the counseling interventions, but also was magnified if the interventions continued over time. Patients in families receiving the interventions remained at home 11 months longer than patients in the control group, and their caregivers were only two-thirds as likely as caregivers in the control group to place them in nursing homes (Mittelman, et al., 1996).

A number of alternative treatments aimed at delaying onset of the symptoms of Alzheimer's disease are also under investigation. There are multi-site, federally funded studies of ginko biloba, an herbal substance, which may help to increase blood flow in the brain, and of certain nonsteroidal anti-inflammatory drugs which may help to reduce the swelling of brain tissue associated with nerve damage in Alzheimer's disease. Also, epidemiological studies of women taking estrogen replacement therapy seemed to show a delay in the onset of Alzheimer's disease (Brenner, et al., 1994). And antioxidants such as vitamin E continue to be examined. Information about other potential "natural" treatments for the symptoms of Alzheimer's disease can be found on the Web site of the National Institutes of Health. Some of these substances can have serious side effects. Before taking any substance for any symptom of memory loss, consult a physician. Specific therapeutic interventions for specific professions will be discussed in later chapters. We would only say here, by way of summary, that some of the best interventions currently available are those which: educate the family caregiver about behavioral management techniques; offer emotional support; engage the person with Alzheimer's in failure-free, therapeutic activities on a daily basis; allow for respite during the week at an Alzheimer adult day health center; modify the home environment to ensure safety and a sense of security; evaluate the person's need for medical treatment, including medications; and monitor the physical and emotional health of both the person with Alzheimer's and the caregiver.

Additionally, some Alzheimer facilities are specifically designed to keep residents as safe and independently functioning as possible. Placement in a therapeutically sound, properly supervised setting such as an Alzheimer's special care unit in a nursing home or an assisted living facility with an Alzheimer's component can be the best intervention for the people with Alzheimer's who are most at risk.

Finally, while there is good reason for optimism about research breakthroughs as to the causes of and cures for Alzheimer's disease, a supervised, structured daily schedule is still the most potent medicine for this disease and for the problem behaviors, such as wandering, which are associated with it. Our shared goal must be to find the best supportive and safe environment for people with dementia.

Credit: The diagnostic specialist table (Table 1.1) and bulleted information on areas of decline are from *Of Two Minds: A Guide to the Care of People With the Dual Diagnosis of Alzheimer's Disease and Mental Retardation* (1996). Reprinted with permission of J. Antonangeli.

CHAPTER 2

Comprehensive Review of the Literature on Wandering Behavior

The term "wandering" is used to describe a common behavioral symptom of Alzheimer's disease and related dementias. The sheer number and variety of definitions used to describe wandering behavior among people with dementia have contributed to a lack of conceptual clarity regarding this common problem.

As a new focus in dementia research, wandering is often studied and written about in broad, general terms. Yet there is a growing body of knowledge about the behavior which can provide a starting point for understanding its intricacies. This chapter presents a solid overview—not an exhaustive listing—of what has been written on the subject. Following a discussion of various definitions of wandering, we will review research findings in the following areas:

- Prevalence rates;
- Costs and consequences;
- Risk factors and possible reasons for the behavior; and
- Recommended management and interventions, including practice-based writings on community and institutional strategies for prevention.

Definitions of Wandering

For two decades, the term "wandering" has been used in research and professional publications to mean a variety of behaviors generally seen in people with Alzheimer's disease or related dementias. However, operational definitions have varied from study to study. Describing the difficulty involved in arriving at a definition for this behavior, the U.S. Veterans Administration, in guidelines published in 1985 for the diagnosis and treatment of dementia, concluded that "wandering was so imprecise as to defy definition, having been applied to behavior as different as pacing, trying doorknobs, entering other people's rooms, talking about 'going home,' attempting to leave or leaving an institution against advice, getting lost on a walk, or simply talking in a way that someone else considers 'disoriented' " (Martino-Saltzman, et al., 1991).

Heim (1986) recognized this definitional problem, and warned against confusing wandering behavior with hyperactivity and pacing, but did not provide a working definition. Table 2.1 at the end of this chapter illustrates that researchers and authors have used the term to refer to an entire continuum of behaviors, including:

1. "the tendency to move about, either in a seemingly aimless or disoriented fashion, in pursuit of an indefinable or unobtainable goal" (Snyder, et al., 1978);
2. "a change in a person's physical location which results in his/her inability to return to the point of origin" (Hussian, 1981);
3. "extended periods of movement without a full awareness of one's behavior" (Namazi, et al., 1989);
4. "pacing, including purposeless wandering" (Cohen-Mansfield & Werner, 1995);
5. "frequent and/or unpredictable pacing with no discernible goal" (Dawson & Reid, 1987);
6. "walking or pacing" (Matteson, et al., 1993);
7. "getting lost outside of the home" (Ballard, et al., 1991; McShane, et al., 1994; Silverstein & Salmons, 1996);
8. "disoriented activities and aimless movements toward undefinable objectives and unobtainable goals" (Monsour & Robb, 1982);
9. "a purposeful behavior that attempts to fulfill a particular need (from the context of the wanderer), is initiated by a cognitively impaired and disoriented individual and is characterized by excessive ambulation that often leads to safety and/or nuisance-related problems" (Thomas, 1995); and
10. "ambulation that is self-initiated and occurs independently of environmental cues" (Coons, 1988).

The Research Literature

As illustrated by the discussion above, the current literature suggests that wandering behavior is widespread, but that the specific scope of the problem is difficult to assess due to differences in the many definitions used to describe it. Differences in research study designs and assessment methods also contribute to the difficulty of pinpointing the prevalence of wandering behavior. Using Table 2.1 as a reference, the following section reviews the research literature concerning those living in the community as well as those living in facilities such as nursing homes. The variables examined by the following studies can be grouped into 3 broad categories:

1. prevalence rates;
2. consequences and related costs of wandering and becoming lost; and
3. risk factors and possible reasons for the behavior, including associated behavioral, situational, and environmental factors.

Prevalence Rates

The Alzheimer's Association estimates that as many as seven out of ten people with Alzheimer's disease or a related dementia will wander off and get lost during the course of the disease, and many of them will do so repeatedly. Calkins and Namazi (1991), surveying family caregivers about home safety modifications, found that 69% of the caregivers indicated that the person in their care had wandered out of the house, making this the most frequently mentioned problem behavior. Hope, Tilling, and Fairburn (1994) report that wandering occurred in 63% of a community sample of people with dementia. Teri, Larson, and Reifler (1988) found that 59% of those with Alzheimer's disease who live in the community wander and become lost. In a study of 463 caregivers, 52% reported that the person with Alzheimer's disease or a related disorder in their care had wandered and become lost and that almost two-thirds of these wanderers were multiple repeat wanderers (Silverstein & Salmons, 1996).

While this behavior is widespread among people with dementia living in the community, the research suggests that it is also common among people with dementia living in long-term care facilities, at least half of whom are estimated to have some form of cognitive impairment such as Alzheimer's disease (Kennedy, 1993). In fact, the majority of studies on wandering have focused their investigations of this behavior on people living in institutions such as nursing homes or assisted living facilities. Data on the size of the wandering problem in these institutions ranges from 11% (Hiatt, 1985) to 24% (Hoffman, et al., 1987; Lucero, Hutchinson, et al., 1993).

Burnside (1981) reports that approximately 20% of the staff in long-term care facilities are aware of at least one incident resulting in the serious injury or death of a wanderer. More precisely, Kennedy writes that each week at least one resident of this nation's nursing home facilities will wander off the premises and die. A study of nursing home elopement insurance claims data reveals that:

1. 70% of elopement claims involve the death of a resident;
2. 45% of elopements occurred within the first 48 hours of admission; and
3. 80% of elopements involved chronic wanderers (Rodriguez, 1993).

Attempts at wandering are also a problem in institutions. In research conducted by Gaffney (1986) in an institutional setting, the author found that over a 15-hour period, a population of 28 wanderers "attempted to leave the unit 457 times and attempted to use an exit 274 times" (pp. 95–96).

Despite the range of prevalence discussed above, many experts agree that all people with dementia should be presumed to be at risk of wandering and becoming lost (Coltharp, et al., 1996; Flaherty & Raia, 1994).

Consequences and Related Costs

The very first consequence of wandering behavior is emotional, both for the people with dementia who wander from a home or institutional setting and become lost, and for their family or professional caregivers, all of whom can be presumed to experience exceptional levels of stress. These episodes may result in serious or fatal injury for the wanderer. Much of the literature asserts that both injury and hospitalization often result as a consequence of unsafe, unsupervised wandering.

Regarding injury, Mayer and Darby (1991, p. 687) cite the "potential for encountering hazards, falls, and fractures" that comes with this problem behavior. Algase (1992, p. 28) points out that "because falls, hip fractures, elopements, deaths, and other hazardous outcomes have long been observed among wanderers, nurses tend to err on the side of caution when dealing with wandering behavior." Finkel (1993, p. 29) concurs, stating that "patients who wander are at risk for injury." Additionally "these individuals are at high risk of dehydration and hypothermia. Their judgment is impaired, their health may be seriously impaired, and they risk experiencing a catastrophic reaction at any time when lost, especially as dark approaches" (Flaherty & Scheft, 1995, p. 7). Furthermore, Sanford (1975) found that wandering "is a prominent cause of hospital admission among dementia sufferers," and in a survey of search and rescue results by Koester and Stooksbury (1995), dementia subjects lost for more than 24 hours suffered a 46% mortality rate. (On the other hand, there were no fatalities among those found within 24 hours.)

Institutionalization is also a frequent consequence, and cost, associated with unmanageable wandering behavior (Ferris, et al., 1987; Finkel, 1993; Kennedy, 1993; Stewart, 1995; Young, et al., 1988). In the Young study, the authors suggest that wandering is one important influence on the decision to institutionalize the person with Alzheimer's disease, and claim that "It is this current lack of knowledge concerning management of such problems as wandering that has forced families to institutionalize the demented patient." It is important to note that, in fact, "It is usually the behavioral problems, rather than the cognitive impairments, that result in the institutionalization of patients with dementing illnesses" (Steele, et al., 1990, p. 1049).

While the research literature discussed above suggests that wandering comes with many risks, Algase (1992, p. 28) also points out that "the actual risk of experiencing a hazardous outcome from wandering is unknown."

Risk Factors and Possible Reasons

Not surprisingly, with the rates of prevalence and the serious consequences, a whole body of research has focused on dementia and wandering behavior. This field has been dominated by studies investigating risk factors. Identifying major characteristics of those who are likely to wander, such studies have had mixed results. Most agree, however, that increased cognitive impairment is a likely risk factor (Algase, 1992; Burns, et al., 1990; Cohen-Mansfield & Werner, 1995; Cooper, et al., 1990; Dawson & Reid, 1987; Logsdon, et al., 1998; Martino-Saltzman, et al., 1991; Teri, et al., 1998).

It indeed appears that levels of impairment are related to incidence of wandering and that as cognitive impairment increases, wandering is more common. The relationship has a peak, however, after which it begins to reverse (Reisberg, et al., 1989). As one might expect, as cognitive impairment approaches late stage and the attendant functional difficulties, wandering is less likely (Franssen, et al., 1993).

Again, because a person in the earliest stage of Alzheimer's disease has a low level of cognitive impairment does not mean that that person will not become lost. Unfortunately, there are just not enough data on wandering behavior among people in this earliest stage to quantify what our experience tells us is indeed a problem, although Rowe and Glover (2001) point out the unpredictability of the behavior even among patients who routinely take walks alone. Moreover, they noted that fewer than 4% of memory-impaired adults who wander away from home are able to return unassisted.

And while it does appear that levels of impairment are related to incidence of wandering, demographic characteristics such as age and gender have not been found to be associated with a higher risk for wandering and becoming lost (Logsdon, et al., 1998; Teri, et al., 1988).

The literature also details various reasons that the behavior occurs. Generally, "the ability of people with Alzheimer's to find their way from one point to another—called 'cognitive mapping'—is impaired very early in the disease process" (Flaherty & Scheft, 1995). Wandering and becoming lost may be:

1. a substitution for social interaction (Monsour & Robb, 1982; Snyder, et al., 1978);
2. an expression of agitation, anxiety, sleep disorder, or unmet physiological needs (Butler & Barnett, 1992; Heim, 1986);
3. a result of boredom, excess energy, lifelong habits, or an attempt to escape crowds or noise (Coons, 1988; Heim, 1986);
4. a result of experiencing fear, seeking exercise or companionship, looking for a childhood home, or trying to get to a former workplace (Flaherty & Raia, 1994).

Summary

Despite the range of prevalence estimates for wandering discussed in this chapter (up to 69%), it is our position that all people with Alzheimer's disease and related dementias who are ambulatory are presumed to be at risk for wandering due to their cognitive deficits, and that one clear standard of incidence might be linked to the degree of cognitive impairment, or stage of the dementia.

Further, there is one description which seems to come closer than any other to an operational definition of wandering, principally, in our view, by capturing the most common and most dangerous characteristics of the behavior:

> Aimless or purposeful motor activity that causes a social problem such as getting lost, leaving a safe environment, or intruding in inappropriate places (Morishita, 1990).

Morishita's definition seems to cover all modes of locomotion, whether by foot or any other means, and all motives, whether aimless or purposeful. As good as it is, however, we have tinkered with it. One assumption is critical to making this definition more appropriate—that the wandering (the "motor activity") is unsupervised. This is a notable distinction, in that there is such a thing in the literature as supervised wandering, which, in fact, can provide both physical exercise and psychological benefit but could conceivably result in someone "leaving a safe environment, or intruding in inappropriate places," even while under supervision. For the purposes of this book, being lost, by definition, means being unsupervised. In the following chapters, wandering means leaving a private residence or care facility of any kind *unsupervised*, and, as Morishita's key phrase emphasizes, "getting lost."

There is another, perhaps semantic distinction to make—that the "environment" does not necessarily have to be "safe," as specified in Morishita's definition. That someone with Alzheimer's who has a roof to live under does not necessarily mean that that person is not alone, malnourished, physically abused, financially exploited, or at risk of burns, falls, or other injury.

We tinkered with Morishita's fine definition for a good reason. The purpose of this book is to enable readers to understand and address a life-threatening behavior—wandering—not as a single event but, as we stated in the *Introduction*, as part of a process. Therefore, we use a definition which cannot confuse the type of wandering we are talking about with any similar but benign behavior. In particular, *there should be no confusion about what has occurred* when the specific wandering "event" triggered by the "process" which led up to it culminates in someone with a dementing illness becoming lost.

Koester has further defined a category of critical wanderer. That is, anyone suffering from dementia who cannot be located by the caregiver due to wandering behavior. Silverstein and Salmons also define wandering along these lines. The following is from Koester (see www.dbs-sar.com) and gives a further indication of the scope of the problem:

> Perhaps one of the best estimates of critical wandering incidents comes from Butler and Barnett (1991). They examined missing person reports from local law enforcement in Arkansas. They reported one critical wanderer per year for every 1,000 persons over the age of 65. Using Evans' estimate of the 10% prevalence of AD among those age 65 or greater, then the incidence of critical wandering is 1% among AD patients. This would suggest that 34,400 critical wandering cases are reported to law enforcement each year in the United States (based on 1998 U.S. Census population estimate). The next number game requires figuring out how many cases of critical wanderers never get reported to law enforcement officials. Silverstein and Salmons contacted by phone 463 caregivers who had registered with the Alzheimer's Association Safe Return Program in eastern Massachusetts.

> They found only 27% of the caregivers reported a missing wanderer to law enforcement. This number also agrees with a study conducted by the Virginia Department of Criminal Justice Services, which contacted caregivers and found that only 34% of the caregivers reported a missing wanderer to law enforcement. These shockingly low numbers are attributed to the caregivers conducting a successful search themselves, calling friends, the subject returns, or that they had never noticed the subject had wandered away in the first place. Using the 1% incident rate reported to law enforcement, the 1998 Census estimate, and the 27% report rate, it appears that 127,400 critical wandering incidents occur each year.

By the year 2040, given Alzheimer's Association estimates of prevalence rates and the aging of the baby-boom generation, this number could grow to over half a million cases each year among a projected Alzheimer's population of 15 million.

This, then, is our operative definition—wherever in the book we say "wandering," we mean:

> Movement by a person with dementia, whether aimless or purposeful, on foot or by other means, which occurs when certain cognitive losses and environmental circumstances intersect, causing that person to become lost in an unsupervised and potentially unsafe setting.

Wandering here always means being lost. And while not all, nor even most, wanderers are reported to police as missing persons, that is nevertheless what they are.

TABLE 2.1 Research Studies That Have Examined Wandering in Alzheimer's Disease or a Related Disorder

Citation	Definition of Wandering	Brief Sample Description: Who Was Included in the Study	Study Question	Selected Findings
Algase (1992b)	2 or more of the following behaviors and designated as wanderer by staff: walks/paces frequently, hyperactive	198 nursing home residents	Differences in cognitive impairment (abstract thinking, language, judgment, spatial skills) among wanderers and nonwanderers.	Wanderers had higher overall levels of cognitive impairment; poorer performance on all 4 cognitive measures.
Ballard, Mohan, Bannister, Handy, & Patel (1991)	Camdex schedule items: getting lost outside the home and getting lost inside the home	92 persons with suspected dementia	Examined problems of getting lost both in and outside the home, and studied the change in prevalence of getting lost with increased cognitive impairment.	Getting lost outside the home was described as a problem in 36.9%, and inside the home in 28.3%; those with Alzheimer's were more likely to get lost outside the home than those with vascular dementia; and there was no correlation between level of cognitive impairment and prevalence of getting lost outside the home.

TABLE 2.1 (continued)

Citation	Definition of Wandering	Brief Sample Description: Who Was Included in the Study	Study Question	Selected Findings
Calkins & Namazi (1991)	Wandered out of the house	59 Alzheimer's caregivers	To identify a variety of modifications made to the home relative to difficult behaviors, to ascertain the effectiveness of these modifications, and to evaluate the impact of the changes on the person and the caregiver.	Sixty-nine percent of the caregivers reported that their family member wandered out of the house (the most frequently mentioned problem); 46 modifications had been made for wandering with 73% of them working well; modifications made included adding dead bolt, chain lock; hanging a curtain in front of door; blocking the door with furniture; and locking the screen door.
Cohen-Mansfield & Werner (1995)	Pacing or purposeless wandering	24 nursing home residents	Environmental conditions present when agitated behaviors occur.	While other agitated behaviors seemed to occur due to discomfort, pacing or purposeless wandering occurred under favorable environmental conditions: normal light, noise, and temperature, during all waking hours, and with high staff levels.

(continued)

TABLE 2.1 ***(continued)***

Citation	Definition of Wandering	Brief Sample Description: Who Was Included in the Study	Study Question	Selected Findings
Cohen-Mansfield, Werner, Marx, & Freedman (1991)	Pacing/wandering	a) 402 nursing home residents b) 6 nursing home residents	Assessed the impact of an in-service training program on nursing home staff's knowledge of dementia, pacing/wandering behavior and management strategies, staff satisfaction, and perceptions of work difficulty and quality of care. Also assessed if changes in staff knowledge impacted the residents or interactions with the residents.	Quiz scores significantly improved immediately following the in-service program but returned to near pretest levels at 1 month follow-up. Residents were allowed to pace/wander to a greater extent at follow-up compared with pretest.
Cooper, Mungas, & Weiler (1990)	Defined as being present if indicated as being present on the neuropsychiatric exam or on a current problem list	680 people with probable Alzheimer's	Relation of cognitive status with abnormal behaviors.	Wandering was associated with a lower MMSE score and increased age. Data supports that wandering is more likely to occur with increasing cognitive loss.

TABLE 2.1 *(continued)*

Citation	Definition of Wandering	Brief Sample Description: Who Was Included in the Study	Study Question	Selected Findings
Crosby, Wyles, Verran, & Tynan (1993)	Escape behaviors—attempting to leave	Qualitative interviews with 11 caregivers	Night behavior of those with Alzheimer's disease.	Many escape behaviors were triggered by environmental stimuli such as a siren or change in light level.
Dawson & Reid (1987)	Frequent and/or unpredictable pacing with no discernible goal	100 nursing home residents identified to be at risk by staff	Factors that differentiate known wanderers from those who had never wandered before	Compared with nonwanderers, wanderers scored higher on two factors: cognitive deficits and hyperactivity.
Groene (1993)	Off-task body movement either by wheelchair or walking that deviated from the group structure. Wandering behavior was determined by on-site health care staff using pedometers, mecury counters, and cyclometers.	30 special care unit residents who had wandered in past		Residents in music groups remained seated or in close proximity longer than those in reading groups.

(continued)

TABLE 2.1 ***(continued)***

Citation	Definition of Wandering	Brief Sample Description: Who Was Included in the Study	Study Question	Selected Findings
Hope & Fairburn (1990)	Investigated as part of the study.	29 patients in the community with dementia who had been classed as "wanderers" by their community psychiatric nurses.	To find the range of behavior which can lead to someone being identified as a "wanderer."	The term "wandering" is used to cover a wide range of very different behaviors and should not be used in the general sense. Instead, the specific behavioral abnormality should be described. Resulting typology includes 1) checking/trailing; 2) pottering; 3) aimless walking; 4) walking directed towards inappropriate purpose; 5) walking directed towards an appropriate purpose, inappropriately frequent; 6) excessive activity; 7) nighttime walking; 8) needs to be brought back home; and, 9) attempts to leave home.

TABLE 2.1 ***(continued)***

Citation	Definition of Wandering	Brief Sample Description: Who Was Included in the Study	Study Question	Selected Findings
Hope, Tilling, & Fairburn (1994)	Investigated as part of the study.	83 patients in the community with dementia	Examined the hypothesis that the different types of wandering behavior form a scale.	Three main categories of wandering behaviors—trying to leave home, being brought back home, and abnormal walking around. The third category can be divided into four subcategories: checking/trailing, increased/aimless walking, pottering, and inappropriate/overappropriate walking.
Klein, Steinberg, Galik, Steele, Sheppard, Warren, Rosenblatt, & Lyketsos (1999)	Wandering behavior in the past two weeks was defined as persistent pacing about and/or persistent attempts to leave a confined area.	638 community-residing new patients with dementia referred for evaluation.	1) provide a profile of patients who wander with respect to dementia characteristics; 2) examine relationship between dementia-associated psychopathology and wandering; and, 3) identify other factors that might impact on wandering such as medical health and the use of psychotropic medication.	Wandering behavior occurred in 17.4% of participants. It was significantly more prevalent in those with Alzheimer Dementia, patients with dementia of longer duration, and patients with more severe dementia. Wandering was associated with moderate to severe depression, delusions, hallucinations, and sleep disorder. Use of neuroleptic medication and male gender were also associated with the behavior.

(continued)

TABLE 2.1 ***(continued)***

Citation	Definition of Wandering	Brief Sample Description: Who Was Included in the Study	Study Question	Selected Findings
Koester & Stooksbury (1995)		Retrospective study of 42 lost dementia of Alzheimer's type (DAT) patients who became the subjects of organized search and rescue efforts in Virginia.	Create a preliminary behavioral profile of lost DAT patients, and determine factors that impact survivability.	Normal elderly individuals on average traveled a greater straight-line distance from point last seen (PLS) than did DAT patients. The mortality rate for DAT patients was 19%. Mortality was caused by hypothermia, dehydration, and drowning. No fatalities were found for DAT patients found within 24 hours. There was a mortality rate of 46% for those requiring more than 24 hours to locate.

TABLE 2.1 (continued)

Citation	Definition of Wandering	Brief Sample Description: Who Was Included in the Study	Study Question	Selected Findings
Lach, Reed, Smith, & Carr (1995)	Self-defined by caregiver answering survey.	35 community-residing persons with Alzheimer's and their caregivers	Determine which safety problems were most common in the populations studied, explore the relationship between dementia severity and safety concerns, and evaluate a home safety instrument.	Wandering was the most common problem, followed by problems with cooking and driving. Many caregivers are practicing some form of safety precautions, they may not be aware of all their options or the best way to prevent problems. For example, wandering was the most common problem but only one family reported using an identification bracelet.
Lucero, Hutchinson, Leger-Krall, & Wilson (1993)		10 patients of a 49-bed special dementia unit; clinical diagnosis of probable Alzheimer's, alert and ambulatory, identified by the nursing staff as someone who exhibits wandering behavior.	Describe wandering behaviors of institutionalized patients with Alzheimer's disease.	The need for interventions is greatest during unstructured periods of the day.

(continued)

TABLE 2.1 ***(continued)***

Citation	Definition of Wandering	Brief Sample Description: Who Was Included in the Study	Study Question	Selected Findings
Marino-Saltzman, Blasch, Morris, & McNeal (1991)	Identified by nursing home staff	40 nursing home residents, 24 of whom were identified by nursing staff as wanderers.	Evaluate patterns of travel of wanderers and nonwanderers; relate engagement in inefficient travel patterns to demographic, psychological, and medical factors.	Four travel patterns were observed: 1) direct travel; 2) lapping; 3) random travel; and, 4) pacing. Travel efficiency was significantly related to cognitive status with inefficient travel most prevalent in severely demented participants.
Monsour & Robb (1982)	Disoriented activities and aimless movements toward undefinable objectives and unattainable goals	22 matched pairs of male wanderers and nonwanderers from the long-term care division of a VA medical center	Why do some elderly people wander while others do not, despite their being similar along other characteristics? Do past psychosocial lifestyles make a difference?	Wanderers had engaged in a higher level of social and leisure activities and had experienced more stressful events prior to their illness.

TABLE 2.1 (continued)

Citation	Definition of Wandering	Brief Sample Description: Who Was Included in the Study	Study Question	Selected Findings
Reed, Lach, Smith, & Birge (1990)		35 caregivers of persons with Alzheimer's disease	Amount of time the person with AD left alone, previous accidents and hazardous behaviors, caregivers' perceptions of the person's safety and need for supervision.	The severity of dementia was highly correlated with the perceived need for supervision and less strongly associated with actual levels of supervision. Hazardous behavior occurring within the past year was most strongly associated with actual supervision.
Richter, Roberto, & Rosenberg (1995)		Focus group interviews with a) 23 family caregivers of persons with AD who were residing in long-term care facilities; b) 22 certified nursing assistants from the same facilities	Sought to identify successful strategies used by family/formal caregivers in communicating with those with AD.	Emergent themes included environmental adjustments and reassurance. Results also suggested that interventions must be individualized and that enhancing the caregivers' skills to deal with problem behaviors may prolong the ability to provide care in the home.

(continued)

TABLE 2.1 ***(continued)***

Citation	Definition of Wandering	Brief Sample Description: Who Was Included in the Study	Study Question	Selected Findings
Rowe & Glover (2001)	Unattended wandering defined as forays into the community without the supervision of a caregiver	Study of 675 missing and discovery incidents reported nationwide to Safe Return over a 13-month period.	Sought to identify patterns of where people were found, how long they had wandered, and how far they had traveled.	Memory-impaired individuals who wander in the community without supervision are at risk of injury or death. About 82% were found within the first 12 hours; about half were found within 5 miles. Most persons were found by good samaritans or law enforcement.

TABLE 2.1 *(continued)*

Citation	Definition of Wandering	Brief Sample Description: Who Was Included in the Study	Study Question	Selected Findings
Salmons (1999)	Wandering and getting lost outside the home	Survey responses of 336 caregivers registered in the Safe Return program of the National Alzheimer's Association; Qualitative interviews with 13 additional caregivers.	Secondary data analysis and qualitative interviewing were used to explore factors influencing supervision provided and precautions taken by caregivers to prevent wandering and getting lost outside the home.	Caregivers were largely aware of the risk of this problem behavior and most took precautions to some extent. Most had experienced wandering and its related problems. Using a higher number of precautions was significantly associated with attempts at wandering and having experienced a serious outcome as a result of a wandering incident. Having experienced wandering was not associated with 24-hour supervision. Being older, being married, having had the diagnosis for a longer period of time, being an older caregiver, and being a caregiver who had participated in a support group were predictors of 24-hour supervision.

(continued)

TABLE 2.1 ***(continued)***

Citation	Definition of Wandering	Brief Sample Description: Who Was Included in the Study	Study Question	Selected Findings
Silverstein & Salmons (1996)	Wandering and getting lost outside the home	463 caregivers registered in the Safe Return program of the national Alzheimer's Association	Provide descriptive data on wandering and getting lost.	Over half had wandered or been lost in the past; most were repeat wanderers. Over 70% were found within one mile of their home with an average missing time period of about 2 hours. Seventy percent reported that a serious consequence/injury resulted from wandering. Over half had been assisted by police for a wandering episode. Twenty percent reported not wearing any identification.

TABLE 2.1 (continued)

Citation	Definition of Wandering	Brief Sample Description: Who Was Included in the Study	Study Question	Selected Findings
Snyder, Rupprecht, Pyrek, Brekhus, & Moss (1978)	A tendency to move about, either in a seemingly aimless or disoriented fashion, or in pursuit of an indefinable or unobtainable goal	16 residents of a Skilled Nursing Facility: 8 whom the staff identified as "wanderers" and 8 nonwanderers	How are wanderers different from nonwanderers? What patterns does the behavior take? What factors seem to prompt wandering?	Wanderers spent more time in motion, had greater involvement in nonsocial behavior, and spent more time in Ritual-Z behavior than nonwanderers. Wanderers did not differ from nonwanderers on sex, marital status, age, or diagnosis of heart disease or stroke. Wanderers had more psychosocial problems, and were more likely to have problems in recent and remote memory, orientation to time and place, and ability to respond appropriately to a given conversation topic. Three types of wandering behavior were identified: 1) overtly goal-directed/searching behavior; 2) overtly goal-directed/industrious behavior; and, 3) apparently nongoal-directed behavior.

(continued)

TABLE 2.1 ***(continued)***

Citation	Definition of Wandering	Brief Sample Description: Who Was Included in the Study	Study Question	Selected Findings
Teri, Larson, & Reifler (1988)	Was one of several behaviors that was rated as being present or absent by a trained geriatric physician	127 persons diagnosed with Alzheimer's disease	The nature of behavioral problems, their rate of occurrence, and their relationship to the disease process	1) Overall, the number of problems increased with increased cognitive impairment, including wandering; this suggests that it is a behavior that is characteristic of the disease, predictable, and should be included in education and intervention programs; 2) the types of problems varied with cognitive severity; and 3) they were not associated with age, gender, duration, or age of onset.

TABLE 2.1 ***(continued)***

Citation	Definition of Wandering	Brief Sample Description: Who Was Included in the Study	Study Question	Selected Findings
Teri, Borson, Kiyak, & Yamagishi (1989)	Tendency to wander off and get lost	56 community-residing persons with Alzheimer's disease	Nature, severity of behavioral problems, relationship to cognitive and functional abilities	The tendency to wander off and get lost occurred more than twice per week in 5% of the caregivers interviewed.
Young, Muir-Nash, & Ninos (1988)	Nocturnal wandering: 1) awake, out of bed, active, and moving; 2) restless while awake	8 persons with Alzheimer's disease with a history of wandering at night	The effect of modified white noise on wandering at night	As a group, the effects of the noise were not significant. Taken individually however, 2 of the participants were significantly less restless and agitated during the noise phase of the study.

CHAPTER 3

The Dementia Wanderer: A Profile

We tend to think of problems happening elsewhere, not to me, not to my community. The less visible the problem is, the more we are able to distance our connection. If there is a message in this book, it is that we hope the reader will see the connection more clearly. So to answer the question, is this a problem for my community? The reader will understand that "yes," it is a problem. Moreover, this problem can and does result in catastrophic consequences.

Such catastrophic consequences were reported by 69% of the caregivers who described wandering episodes in Silverstein and Salmon's 1996 study. The caregivers shared accounts of individuals who were found in snow embankments or in wooded areas; and still others who returned home badly bruised. Rader, Doan, and Schwab (1985) reported that 20 to 25% of the nursing home staff they surveyed knew of a serious injury or death of a confused elderly person, likely due to wandering. Koester and Stooksbury (1995) reported that the majority of wanderers in their study were found in drainages/creeks or heavy brush/briars (p. 38). These observations led them to formulate a "following a path of least resistance" or "pinball" hypothesis. In other words, going until you get stuck. Another way to think of this phenomenon is the carnival ride, "bumper car," where the car moves in a straight line until it hits another car and then changes direction.

Wandering in the News

It rarely makes the front page, but news about missing elders quite often appears in a brief clipping further into the paper. These are hardly ever the feature stories. We hear of these incidents on television or radio or read human interest stories and think, "too bad" or "how sad." We may even think, "There is nothing that could have been done." Well, we believe that there is a lot that can be done.

Taken one at a time, the incidents seem isolated—but viewing them together as you will see in the accounts that follow, the reader is bound to feel the same sense of urgency felt by the authors of the need for greater recognition of wandering behavior as a concern for all communities. We will start by presenting the back page or "filler" stories to you in a way that illustrates that the larger story has yet to be told.

It is important to underscore that Alzheimer's disease and its related disorders impact individuals across all socioeconomic and demographic strata, and therefore the risk of dangerous wandering episodes exists across all geographic boundaries. The following are examples of actual reports that appeared during 1997 to 2000 in newspapers across the nation. A simple Lexis-Nexis search with keywords "wandering" and "Alzheimer's" will generate a similar listing if the reader is interested in an update.

Here are examples where individuals were found too late:

- In January 1997, the Milwaukee Journal Sentinel reported that the body of a 65-year-old woman with Alzheimer's disease was found in a state park after being missing for 3 days.
- In February 1997, the New Orleans Times told of a 91-year-old man with Alzheimer's disease who was found dead on the grounds of a funeral home 8 days after he failed to return home from visiting relatives. Police found his car, out of gas, on Interstate 49 but there was no clue as to how he got from the car to the area where he was found.
- In August 1997, the Times-Picayune mentioned that a decomposed body found in a field near the New Orleans International Airport might be that of a woman with Alzheimer's disease who disappeared from her daughter's home 3 weeks previously.

The next year featured more deaths:

- In January 1998, the Evansville Courier reported that an 80-year-old woman suspected of having Alzheimer's disease was found dead from hypothermia a quarter of a mile from her home after having been missing for 3 days.

- Later that month, the St. Petersburg Times mentioned the skeletal remains of a 70-year-old man with Alzheimer's disease that were found by a survey crew. He had been missing for 5 months.
- The San Francisco Chronicle told of an 80-year-old woman with diabetes and Alzheimer's disease found dead in a creek four blocks from where she was last seen.
- In February 1998, the Times-Picayune noted that after being reported missing from a nursing home just 1 hour earlier, the body of a woman was found three blocks away floating in 6 to 8 feet of water in a canal. It was believed that she became disoriented and accidentally drowned.
- Also in February 1998, the New York Daily News reported that a van driver struck and killed an elderly man wandering along the Cross Bronx Expressway. It was unclear why he was walking on the expressway, but the police source said his family told the police that he may have been disoriented because of Alzheimer's.
- In April 1998, the San Francisco Chronicle mentioned that a 79-year-old man with Alzheimer's disease was found dead next to a fence in Sacramento's River Park area 10 days after his disappearance.
- Also in April 1998, the Virginia-Pilot and the Ledger-Star reported that the body of an 81-year-old man who suffered from Alzheimer's disease was found in a lake near his home after he had been missing for 2 days.
- In May 1998, the St. Petersburg Times reported that the body of a 60-year-old man who had Alzheimer's disease was found floating in a cypress swamp 2 days after he had wandered away from an assisted living center.
- In May 2000, the Pittsburgh Post Gazette reported that an 84-year-old woman with Alzheimer's disease was found dead after wandering away 2 days earlier from a personal care center. The article noted that the woman had had a history of walking away from caretakers. Her body was found on a hillside behind an industrial plant. The coroner noted that this was the third or fourth situation that year in which an elderly person had eloped from a nursing home and ultimately died.

Not all of the news stories are reports about deaths. Some individuals have been found alive. These occurrences should be viewed as warnings or "wake-up calls" to communities and care providers. Family members and professional care providers must learn to recognize that unless the situations that enabled the individual to wander away in the first place are altered, the individual is still at risk of the consequences of a dangerous wandering episode. That point was made very clear in the Silverstein and Salmons (1996) study when a caregiver told them, "He (the person with dementia) does not have a problem with wandering. The police bring him home every time!" When asked how many times the police had brought her husband home, the caregiver replied, "about ten times." In another example, a husband who worked full time was unaware that his wife wandered until a neighbor called him at work to let him know—apparently, the neighbors would always direct her home but this time they could not find her. Thus, even well-meaning professionals and friends may act as "enablers" to a potentially dangerous situation rather than provide effective intervention.

Here are examples reported in the newspapers that should serve as serious warnings:

- In January 1997, the Daily Oklahoman reported that a 66-year-old man with Alzheimer's disease who had walked away from his home 3 days before was found at a bar.
- Also in January 1997, the Baton Rouge Advocate noted that a 72-year-old woman with Alzheimer's disease survived two nights of cold temperatures after she walked away from her home. A logger found her.
- Finally, in late January 1997, the Grand Rapids Press mentioned that a 73-year-old man with Alzheimer's disease was found in the Interstate 96 median 5 hours after he wandered away from a health care facility.
- In July 1997, the Atlanta Constitution reported that a 75-year-old woman with Alzheimer's disease wandered away from a personal care home and spent the night outdoors before police found her the next day. She was wearing only a blue nightgown. She was spotted by a police helicopter in a patch of flowers in a wooded area near the facility. The administrator commented that the woman had walked away at a time of day when shifts were changing.
- In October 1997, the Chicago Tribune reported that an 83-year-old man with Alzheimer's disease who had been missing for 2 days was found unharmed asleep in a sleeping bag alongside railroad tracks. He had wandered away from a senior citizen day care program.
- In November 1997, the Tucson Citizen mentioned that a 61-year-old woman with Alzheimer's disease was found under a tree behind a fast food restaurant after being missing for 3 days.
- Later in November, 1997, the Boston Herald reported that a Massachusetts man who had Alzheimer's disease was found wandering the streets of Miami 1 day after he was declared missing by Massachusetts relatives. The police found him and took him to be checked out at a

hospital where a nurse recognized him from a photo that appeared on the news. Apparently, he had boarded the wrong connecting flight in Atlanta after visiting relatives.

- In December 1997, the San Diego Union-Tribune told about a 70-year-old man with Alzheimer's disease who was found sitting in his car about 50 miles away from his home a day after he was reported missing.
- Also in December 1997, the San Diego Union-Tribune noted that a 72-year-old man with Alzheimer's disease was found after being missing for 8 days. He apparently hitchhiked to Spokane, Washington and told officers that he was headed to Idaho.

More of the same type of incidents were found in the next year:

- In January 1998, the Baltimore Sun reported that a 70-year-old man with Alzheimer's disease who had been missing for 12 hours was found wandering in a neighboring county after a search involving six government agencies.
- In March 1998, the San Francisco Chronicle mentioned that an 85-year-old man with Alzheimer's disease who was missing for 2 days was found safe in a gully behind a racetrack. He had gone to the racetrack with his family but became separated from them.
- In May 1998, the Providence Sunday Journal reported an 87-year-old woman with Alzheimer's disease was found in the woods near Rhode Island College by campus police. She was wearing pajamas and was wet and cold.
- Later in May 1998, the Des Moines Register reported that the police were looking for an Alzheimer's patient, age 86, who was missing over 24 hours. (A second article indicated that they had found him 2 days later, unharmed, a few blocks away from his home.)
- Also in May 1998, the Tulsa World reported that a 72-year-old woman with Alzheimer's disease was found in an abandoned warehouse 2 days after she wandered away from her home.
- In June 1998, the Buffalo News reported that a 57-year-old woman who suffered from Alzheimer's disease was found about 24 hours after she left home to walk her dog. Television broadcasts of the woman's description and a photograph provided the break in the case. Some people saw her on the news and flagged police down.
- In October 2000, the Boston Globe reported a story about a 96-year-old woman with Alzheimer's disease who had been lost for 3 days. She was found sitting in a pile of leaves with her back against a tree

in a wooded wetland area a quarter of a mile from her home. She was tired, cold, and confused. Local police said that she had wandered off before.

This next report highlights concern regarding the issue of elder abuse and neglect. Caregivers may use means to prevent wandering that could be harsh and cruel. Reaching the caregiver before he or she has exhausted all personal strategies for coping with unsafe wandering may not only help the caregiver but also prevent potential abuse.

- In June 2000, the Milwaukee Journal Sentinel reported how police found an 83-year-old woman with Alzheimer's disease tied with a wire to a door hinge in her apartment by her 53-year-old son, apparently to keep her from wandering away. She had a 10- to 12-foot-long wire looped around her waist and held together with a padlock. The wire was long enough for her to get to the bathroom and to the kitchen but when the police found her, she was all tangled up. Her son told police that for the last several weeks he has had problems with the woman wandering away. Neighbors said that they had not seen the woman for 3 weeks.

Then there are the notices regarding people who are still missing:

- In February 1997, the Montreal Gazette wrote about an 86-year-old woman with Alzheimer's disease who lives alone and was reported missing a day earlier by an acquaintance who checks on her daily. She was reported walking along the highway but police had yet to locate her.
- In May 1997, the Boston Herald reported that the police continued searching for a 77-year-old man with Alzheimer's disease who had wandered away from his home the day before. It was the second time that week that he was missing.
- In September 1997, the St. Petersburg Times reported that the Sheriff's Office was seeking help in locating a 70-year-old man who wandered away from a care facility 2 weeks prior. The man was in the early stages of Alzheimer's disease, had little short-term memory, and needed to take medication.
- In October 1997, the St. Louis Post-Dispatch mentioned that a 61-year-old diabetic man with Alzheimer's disease who was reported missing after 1 day by his wife who returned home and found his car gone. She became concerned when he did not show up for his tee time at his golf club.

- In November 1997, the Boston Globe wrote about a 73-year-old man with Alzheimer's disease who was reported missing and was last seen near a reservoir. Relatives said that he had wandered away from home several times but that it was the first time he had been gone overnight.

The year 1998 brought more of the same:

- In April 1998, the Richmond Times reported that police were still searching for a 71-year-old man with Alzheimer's disease who drove away from his home 4 days earlier.
- In May 1998, the Providence Journal-Bulletin noted that police were still continuing their search for an 87-year-old woman with Alzheimer's disease who disappeared 2 days earlier.

These news stories illustrate the prevalence of this phenomenon nationwide. The words in the above news clippings vividly illustrate the similar pattern that begins to emerge around wandering: *woods, water, driving, living alone, nursing home or day center, found nearby.* In addition, the subtle denial by family members who know the diagnosis but do not accept the potential for serious consequences also comes through in these clippings: *did not show up for his golf game, did not return home from driving to see relatives, became separated from his family at a racetrack, second time this week, first time he's been gone overnight.*

Law enforcement, family, and professional care-providers are well aware that wandering is a behavior that can have serious consequences. We would argue that by the time it makes the news, the situation is already out of control. It is likely that many of the individuals who make it to the newspapers have wandered or attempted to wander before. They were either found by family members, friends, or neighbors, or prevented from wandering off in the first place. In fact, several of the articles did allude to a history of wandering behavior. Remember, Alzheimer's is a disease that typically lasts from 8 to 15 years from the time of first symptoms. The individual with dementia may be giving the caregiver warnings early on in the disease process, but those warnings may go unheeded. If we are not looking for clues, we will not see them.

A Profile of Who Is Likely to Wander

Is it possible to provide a profile of the individual who is likely to wander? Family caregivers would like to know if wandering is a problem behavior they are likely to encounter. The simple answer is "yes." Author Gerald Flaherty has said, "If an individual with Alzheimer's disease can walk, he or she will wander at some stage during the disease process." Professional caregivers want to be prepared with behavior management strategies. Law enforcement officers would like to know if patterns of elopement are predictable so that they can more effectively plan their searches. There is no cookbook response. There are, however, observations that may be gleaned from research and best practice.

As already stated, if the person with dementia is mobile, the risk of wandering should be taken seriously. Caregivers erroneously assume that if it has not happened in the past, it will not happen in the future. Caregivers are also deluged with recommendations—both from professionals and from family and friends. Caregiving for an individual with Alzheimer's disease can last many years; some recommendations just do not seem relevant for the moment. Just as the caregiver who does not follow the professional precautionary recommendation to put locks on cabinets below the kitchen sink learns too late that her family member will, indeed, swallow bleach (Silverstein, Hyde, & Ohta, 1993), caregivers should anticipate that wandering will occur.

Salmons (1999) provides some insight into a caregiver's experiences with a family member who wanders by reporting a qualitative account of a first episode:

> One day a friend called and said, "Do you realize he's on the bus going to [the city]?" And I said, "No." So he was gone all day, and what he said when he was brought home (by a friend who spotted him) was that someone owed him $800,000. This was at 7:00 a.m. and he had been gone since two in the afternoon. It was perfectly normal for him, as far as he was concerned, that he do [sic] that.

Are there personality traits or circumstances that may trigger wandering behavior? Salmons (1999) provides some caregiver accounts that suggest that there may be some predisposing factors.

- **Fear or Hallucinations.** She said somebody was chasing her, somebody was after her and she had not a clue where she was.
- **Personality or Lifelong Habits.** He never liked to be confined. He wanted to be out all the time. So by taking the car away from him and then by putting him in the condo, I knew I could only keep him in so long. So everyday we'd take a ride and go down to the [city] just to keep him out and keep him moving. He liked to walk.

- **Going Home.** She always wanted to go home—she had to go home to see her mother. We would constantly say, "this is your home, see here's all your things, here's all the paintings that Dad did." Lots of times she would think that all her things were here and how did they ever get here? She's lived here for 22 years but she still thinks home is [city] or someplace that she lived long before this.
- **On a Mission.** She loves cats. She didn't have one at the time but a neighbor did—she heard the cat outside and she went out in the street in her pajamas to try to get the cat.
- **Clothing is Likely To Be Inappropriate for the Weather.** At first, I didn't realize that she would do that but she walked—in December—she walked out of the house in her slippers and bathrobe and walked down the street—trying to get back to New York City [they were living in Cape Cod, Massachusetts at the time].

In fact, Silverstein and Salmons (1996) reported that many of the accounts of individuals whom caregivers reported on in their study were found dressed in sleeping apparel—nightgowns and slippers; or in clothing that was not appropriate for the weather—heavily layered in summer or light sweaters in winter. Others wore their underwear over their outer clothing.

What Does the Research Tell Us?

According to Teri, Larson, and Reifler (1988), 69% of individuals with dementia are wanderers. The great majority of these individuals are likely to live in the community either with their relatives (75–80%) or alone (20+%). Institutionalized settings such as nursing homes, assisted living residences, and adult day health care facilities are not necessarily safe havens for wanderers. As noted in chapter 1, data regarding the prevalence of institutionalized dementia patients who wander from nursing homes range from estimates of 11% (Hiatt, 1985) to 24% (Hoffman, et al., 1987). In the Silverstein and Salmons (1996) community-based study, 52% had wandered. Moreover, Silverstein and Salmons emphasize that those who had wandered were likely to have done so multiple times. In fact, 72% of those who had wandered or been lost, did so on repeated occasions. Koester and Stooksbury (1992) confirm that persons found by Virginia Search and Rescue who had Alzheimer's disease were likely to have wandered before. Caregivers of those who had not actually wandered away in the Silverstein and Salmons study were fearful that they might in the future, in that 79% of these caregivers reported that the individual with dementia had tried to leave but was stopped in time.

What Are Some of the Traits Reported in the Literature?

Tetewsky and Duffy (1999) report that motion blindness may be one reason so many people with Alzheimer's disease wander and become lost in familiar places. According to Tetewsky and Duffy (1999), motion blindness is an impairment of optic flow—the inability to process the complex flow of information a patient's eyes take in as they move through the environment. Tetewsky and Duffy explain that while the normal view of the world is a motion-filled, movie-like environment, the world for some people with Alzheimer's disease appears to be a series of still frames, like a strobe where the intermediate steps are missing. In an unexpected and potentially significant finding, Tetewsky and Duffy (1999) discovered that several of the subjects in their study who had no apparent memory loss nevertheless tested abnormally for motion blindness, and later on went on to develop probable Alzheimer's disease. The researchers believe that motion blindness may precede memory loss in some people with Alzheimer's and may be useful as an early indicator for identifying individuals who may be at increased risk for wandering.

Are There Behaviors That Separate the Wanderer From the Nonwanderer?

Much has been learned from research on nursing home populations. Hall and colleagues (1995) reports that patients who are anxious tend to wander more. She suggests that anxious behaviors occur along with feelings of stress. Monsour and Robb (1982) found that nursing home patients who wandered engaged in a higher level of social and leisure activities. Snyder and colleagues (1978) also referred to longitudinal or historical psychological factors that may influence the tendency to wander: (1) lifelong patterns of coping with stress such as taking a brisk walk or a long stroll; (2) previous work roles; and (3) searching for security. Wanderers express a need to be somewhere and experience stress when they are blocked from getting there.

Companion behaviors to wandering noted by Teri and colleagues (1988) were problems with personal hygiene, agitation, and incontinence. In 1978, Snyder and colleagues observed that wanderers were more likely to exhibit nonsocial behavior, that is, behavior that occurs alone and not directly or indirectly oriented to others (p. 273). Dawson and Reid (1987) reported three factors that were significant to research on wandering: cognitive deficits, agitation/aggression, and hyperactivity. Dawson and Reid (1987) further profile the wanderer as distinguished from the nonwanderer, as an individual with greater difficulties with speech, reading, incontinence, constant rather than transitory disorientation, and the inability to know when they are lost. Further, they also exhibit better social skills, better hearing, are less withdrawn, and are quite mobile insofar as they have a good gait and are seemingly perpetually active (p. 106).

Algase (1999) offers a Need-Driven Dementia Compromised Behavior (NDB) Model where wandering is presumed to result from the interplay of background and proximal factors. The background factors include psychosocial and demographic variables. The proximal factors are physiological, psychological, social, and environmental factors that can change. Algase suggests that people with dementia who wander have poorer neurocognitive abilities and declining language skills that affect one's ability for social engagement. Algase concludes that wandering may emerge to fill the void. Algase offers explanations about five neurocognitive deficits and discusses the implication of each deficit:

- Memory and attention deficits—the individual may be unable to keep a destination in mind and forget where they are going. He or she is unable to sort relevant from nonessential information.
- Visual-spatial deficits—the individual may know the destination but not how to get there. He or she may feel lost or afraid.
- Perseveration—the individual may be unable to stop, even when approaching the intended destination.
- Excessive motor activity—the individual is compelled to walk even more than he or she desires.
- Expressive language deficits—the individual has difficulty in expressing needs, desires, and intentions (Algase, 1999, p. 13).

Klein and colleagues (1999) observed in their study of 638 community-residing persons with dementia that persons who were diagnosed with Alzheimer's disease were significantly more likely to wander than those who were diagnosed with vascular dementia or any other dementia. The probability of wandering increased significantly with the increasing severity of the dementia. Moderate to severe depression, delusions, hallucinations, and sleep disorders were all significantly more frequent in wanderers than nonwanderers. Klein and colleagues also examined sociodemographic variables in their study and although earlier studies had not found significant associations between behavioral problems (wandering included) and an individual's gender (Teri, et al., 1988), Klein and colleagues did find significant associations. Specifically, male gender and the concurrent use of neuroleptic medication were associated with the likelihood of wandering. Klein and colleagues confirmed earlier studies that did not find significant relationships between age, race, education, caregiver identity, general medical health, or the use of antidepressant or anxiolytic medications.

Is Anyone Watching?

The lack of supervision is likely to be the major reason that persons with dementia will wander. There are times, in fact, when some individuals with dementia are left unsupervised. About 40% of the wanderers in the Silverstein and Salmons (1996) study were left to go out by themselves at least some of the time, while 26% were left to come and go as they please. For these caregivers, the potential that the individual with dementia would wander away and become lost was not perceived as a likely risk. Caregivers are often faced with judgment calls and may not possess the knowledge and experience to exercise best judgment when it comes to dementia care. One caregiver intentionally sent her husband out for a walk to give herself a needed break. Other caregivers were employed and learned from neighbors that their family members were continuously being returned after becoming lost in the community. Still other caregivers thought that leaving the individual locked in the car during a trip to the mall would be safe, only to return to an empty car.

When Do They Wander?

While wandering episodes were reported to occur at all times of day and during every season of the year, the afternoon to early evening hours during the spring and summer months yielded a higher frequency of occurrence in the Silverstein and Salmons study. This study was conducted in Massachusetts and may not be generalizable to other states with warmer climates. Snyder and colleagues (1978) observed that wandering increased during the first days of warm weather, after a cold or wet spell, during extreme changes in atmospheric pressure, or even with a full moon (p. 279). Algase (1999) in distinguishing between direct and random wandering, states that random wandering, the most common pattern of wandering, increases in frequency and duration as the day goes on, while direct wandering is more frequent earlier in the day. Crosby and colleagues (1993) cited nighttime wandering as a trigger for institutionalization. Time of day can impact a caregiver's ability to cope with and manage a difficult behavior.

Most Wanderers Do Not Travel Very Far

Seventy percent of those who wandered in the Silverstein and Salmons study were found one mile or less from their residence/starting point. Flaherty (1996) estimates that most wanderers will be found within a mile and a half radius of their home. Koester and Stooksbury (1995) confirm that once an individual with dementia becomes lost, he is usually found close to the PLS (point last seen) (p. 40).

An explanation for the relatively short distance traveled is offered by Visser (1983) whose study on gait and balance in patients with senile dementia revealed a shorter step length, lower gait speed, lower stepping frequency, greater step-to-step variability, and greater sway path.

How Do They Travel?

While the great majority of wanderers will merely walk away from their residence, others are likely to drive, take the bus, hail a taxi, hitchhike, or ride the subway or train. Most lost Alzheimer's patients were on foot (almost 90% in the 1996 Silverstein & Salmons study and 84% in the 2001 Rowe & Glover study). Fifteen percent of the wanderers in the Silverstein and Salmons study were lost while driving (as were almost 6% in the 2001 Rowe study). When probed, caregivers would admit that they did not feel safe with the individual driving but that they could not take away his or her independence. Other caregivers, particularly spouses who did not drive, relied on the individual with dementia for their own transportation.

Salmons (1999) shares the following caregiver's account of driving with a person with dementia.

> When I first noticed that something was wrong, we had gone for a ride and we ended up in [a town he knew well]. He stopped the car, he was driving, and he said that he didn't know where he was, he was lost. I said, "Why don't we just stay here for a while until it comes back?" And we sat for about a half hour until it came back.

Driving is a complex activity that necessitates the kinds of quick reactions, clear sensory abilities, and split-second decisions that become increasingly difficult for someone with Alzheimer's disease. Recognizing that there is a greater prevalence of Alzheimer's disease among older adults, it is relevant to inform our discussion by looking at the research on older drivers. Older drivers are not only more likely to experience an increased accident rate per mile driven, but they are also have a greater risk of dying in that automobile accident (Cobb & Coughlin, 1997; Gillespie & McMurdok, 1999; Miller & Morley, 1993; Johansson, Bronge, Lundberg, Persson, Seideman, & Viitanen, 1996; Sims, Owsley, Allman, Ball, & Smoot, 1998). The question now becomes the choice between personal well-being and the protection of others. "Once the question of competence to operate an automobile has been raised, ethical dilemmas must be addressed regarding the benefit of continued driving for the individual versus the risk to that person and society as a whole" (Reuben, Silliman, & Traines, 1988).

Adler (1997) reported that dementia may compromise the competence and safety of an older driver. Persons with dementia frequently experience disturbances in memory, language, orientation, visual-spatial skills, and the ability to perform complex tasks. Individuals may become lost on familiar streets, fail to follow directional signs, and drive at inappropriate speeds.

A 1997 Scandinavian study examined the brains of elderly car-crash victims and found that a third showed clear evidence of early Alzheimer's disease (Johansson, Bogdanovic, Kalimo, Winblad, & Viitanen, 1997).

Family members differ in their desires and abilities to address concerns related to the older driver. Revealing and reporting impaired drivers is often a difficult task for family members. This is especially problematic if the impaired driver is the only driver in the household (Kapust, 1992). "Family members have enough to cope with as the older person declines and should not have to serve as the judge in assessing the ability to drive and as the enforcer in setting driving limits" (Gillins, 1990). Even in situations where a family member wishes to confront his or her loved one, it may be easier to do so if it is not a solo mission. The family member may have a better time saying "the doctor" or "the state says you shouldn't drive," rather than, "I don't think you should be driving" (Gillins, 1990).

Shemon and Christensen (1991) report that all too often, the driving issue is not addressed by the family or a health care team member until the patient is involved in an accident or gets lost when driving alone. Shemon and Christensen noted a 1988 study of 53 dementia caregivers by Lucas-Blaustein, Filipp, Duncan, and Tune where 30% reported that the individual with dementia continued to drive with 80% of them driving alone at times and 44% regularly getting lost while driving (p. 5). In their own 1991 study of 64 individuals with dementia, Shemon and Christensen learned that memory problems were the primary reason given for individuals who had discontinuing driving. Those individuals who were still driving (15 people) were given a road examination. The researchers observed the following driving errors during the road test:

- Incomplete stops at stop signs;
- Not utilizing signals or checking blind spots;
- Not keeping the car in the proper lane;
- Improper lane changes;
- Driving too fast for existing conditions;
- Wide right turns;
- Difficulty understanding road signs; and
- Improper use of gas and brake pedals.

None of the study participants successfully completed the road examination. Shemon and Christensen concluded that until more data are available, it is better to err on the side of overcautiousness regarding the issue of driving and Alzheimer's disease. They recommended that all individuals with Alzheimer's disease who are currently driving should be given a complete driving evaluation. Freedman and Freedman (1996) further specify that given the current level of knowledge, patients with mild to severe cognitive decline should drive only with someone else in the car who functions as a "copilot" and when Alzheimer's disease is definitely diagnosed, the individual should cease driving (p. 877).

Stutts (1998) questioned whether older drivers themselves restrict their own driving. She found clear patterns of reduced driving. Lower cognitive and visual functioning were closely associated with "lower annual miles and greater avoidance of high-risk driving situations." Although it is reassuring to know older drivers as a whole may restrict their own driving, this does not mean that all impaired drivers reduce their driving exposure (Stutts, 1998).

Silverstein and Murtha (2001) report that states are quite varied in their policies with regard to license renewal practices and professional obligation to report unsafe driving. The decision about when to stop driving is a highly charged one, particularly when alternative forms of transportation are unavailable, inaccessible, or undesirable. Currently, the responsibility for identifying impaired drivers varies with law enforcement, family members, or physicians—if that responsibility is assumed by anyone at all. Law enforcement officers as well as state departments of motor vehicles are the only preventive measures in place.

The group most often thought to be in charge of identifying potentially problematic drivers is physicians, even though there is no specific protocol in line for them to rely upon. Mandatory reporting as in protective service cases does not exist. Many researchers (Miller & Morley, 1993; Reuben, et al., 1988) note Medical Advisory Boards as systems set in place to assist physicians in interacting with state authorities. The American Medical Association changed its ethical guidelines in 1999 to let doctors notify the Department of Motor Vehicles in their states of patients with medical conditions that could make them unsafe drivers. Specifically, the new policy makes public safety a priority over the confidentiality of patients with medical conditions such as senile dementia or alcoholism (Associated Press, 12/8/99).

Much research has been done in an attempt to decipher the role that physicians are to play according to the law. In a study by Miller and Morley (1993) several physicians were unaware of the American Medical Association's guidelines for physician reporting. Many felt that it was their responsibility, but over 60% admitted that they had never referred a patient for driving evaluation. Less than one third of the physicians questioned in the Miller and Morley (1993) study actually kept records of their patients' driving status. Another question raised with regard to physicians in the literature on driving is whether reporting unsafe drivers should actually be the physicians' responsibility at all. There is research to suggest that the impairments associated with unsafe driving are not visible through a routine physical examination. Purely clinical examinations possess little value in evaluating driving ability. It is in using cognitive rating scales and performance tests that cognitive impairments are revealed (Johansson, et al., 1996). However, it is also hard for physicians to make judgments that correspond to on-road errors based on office examinations (Kapust, 1999).

The litmus test we offer to family members or other care providers who are concerned about the driving issue but have yet to take any action to address it, consists of two questions:

1. Would you feel comfortable having your child be a passenger in a car driven by the individual with dementia?
2. Would you feel comfortable having your child cross the street in front of a car driven by the individual with dementia?

If the answer to either of these questions is "No," then it is time to actively take steps to monitor this concern. Two actions that can be taken may help the individual, him or herself, reach the conclusion to stop driving.

- Individuals with Alzheimer's disease should have their driving skills periodically reevaluated with an assessment that includes a road test.

- Individuals with Alzheimer's disease should not drive alone. The passenger must be able to assume the active role of copilot—offering directional assistance, if needed.

Summary

We are asking that family and professional care providers pay attention to wandering behavior. Any mobile person with dementia is a potential wanderer. Keep these principles in mind:

- There are few safe havens
- Wandering should be anticipated
- Wandering is a repetitive behavior

Hallmark behaviors or cognitive/medical circumstances:

- Anxiety
- Moderate to severe depression
- Delusions
- Hallucinations
- Sleep disorders

Other contributing circumstances:

- Concurrent use of neuroleptic medication
- Dressed inappropriately for the weather
- Lifelong patterns of coping with stress, such as taking a brisk walk or a long stroll
- Previous work roles
- Lack of supervision

Part II

Current Community Responses to Wandering Behavior: What Works, What Doesn't, and Why

Introduction

Considering its prevalence and the associated risks to the wanderer—not to mention the tremendous stress for family and professional caregivers discussed in earlier chapters, it is not surprising that wandering behavior has become a focus in dementia research. Work related to the behavior has largely been dominated by studies investigating risk factors, possible reasons for the behavior, and types of strategies which might be used to prevent it. While this previous research has imparted some invaluable insight, little is known about caregivers' actions, concerns, and perceptions about the behavior and its risks.

Surveying 59 family caregivers about home safety modifications, Calkins and Namazi (1991) found that "approximately two-thirds (69%) of the caregivers indicated their family member wandered out of the house, making this the most frequently mentioned problem" (p. 26). What we know from this and other literature on wandering behavior is that while most caregivers are aware of the risk of wandering and most do take some precautions, many still do not regard the behavior as a serious problem. More to the point, the overall caregiver and community response to incidents of people with dementia wandering and becoming lost is limited, uneven, and often inappropriate. Current responses, across the board, are far more crisis-oriented than preventive, whether initiated by family and professional caregivers, by law enforcement and related agencies such as search and rescue organizations, or even by manufacturers of safety and alarm devices.

And while caregivers have become quite resourceful and well-meaning in responding to wandering behavior, they sometimes choose precautionary steps which may themselves be problematic, such as locking the person with dementia in the home or in the car while the caregiver shops. As for the community response, local police may be continually recovering the lost person with dementia and bringing him or her home, and the person's neighbors doing the same thing, all without any referral to the formal elder service network which, for its part, may be ignoring the full extent of the risk even when such a referral is made. This collective response may even enable the wanderer to continue a high-risk behavior.

We will first examine current responses among family caregivers, not only to guide them in decision-making for the memory-impaired person in their care, but as a guide for professionals who work with these families on issues of patient safety. We will then move on to discuss responses among other categories of professionals, describing current management strategies as we go, with the help of direct quotes from caregivers about their experiences with wandering behavior and their attitudes and opinions about this issue. In succeeding chapters in part III aimed at specific categories of caregivers, providers and other professionals, we will elaborate on recommended strategies for managing the behavior.

CHAPTER 4

The Caregiver

Understanding influential factors is key to helping caregivers deal with the difficulties wandering behavior presents, to reduce its frequency, and to minimize its consequences. What influences caregivers' use of precautions to prevent unsafe wandering? For example, do caregiver practices concerning wandering behavior reflect their experiences with this problem?

We will attempt here to convey a more complete understanding of what family caregivers feel and do about the problem of wandering, and how they estimate risk in order to act protectively. We will identify strategies and underlying thoughts regarding safety and protection, notwithstanding significant issues of autonomy and quality of life.

Influences on Use of Precautions and Levels of Supervision

While the existing literature does not empirically explore the factors that influence caregivers' use of precautions and supervision for wandering, it does suggest that even though those with dementia have a high risk of wandering and getting lost, many caregivers may not be aware of that risk or the precautions that can be taken. Social learning theory suggests that we learn through direct consequences (Bandura, 1973; Grusec, 1992). Experiencing wandering behavior and its seriousness should, and for the most part does, lead caregivers to take greater precautions. However, not all caregivers regard this behavior as a serious problem. Nor are experiences with wandering necessarily associated with around-the-clock supervision.

In her 1999 study, Salmons started with three hypotheses:

1. that those who view wandering as a problem are likely to take more precautions to prevent this behavior;
2. that caregivers who have experienced wandering episodes or attempts are likely to take more precautions to prevent this behavior; and
3. that the nature of wandering experiences has an influence on caregiver practice.

What she discovered was somewhat surprising:

- considering wandering to be a problem *was not* associated with using a greater number of precautions;
- caregivers of people who have wandered or gotten lost in the past *did not* use a significantly greater number of precautions, even if they had experienced wandering directly.

Less surprising, in examining the third hypothesis, she found that some characteristics of wandering experiences *were* associated with using more precautions. More specifically, trying to leave home a greater number of times and experiencing a serious consequence as a result of a wandering episode were significantly associated with using more precautions.

Caring for a person who often tries to leave the home unsupervised and caring for a person who has experienced a serious consequence as a result of a wandering episode are salient events that are likely to affect caregivers' actions. Caregivers of those who had ever tried to leave home and those who had tried to leave home a greater number of times tended to use a greater number of precautions for this behavior. While this relationship between attempts at wandering and number of precautions was logically expected and grounded in the literature (Hall, et al., 1995), Salmons found it interesting that *attempts* to wander appeared to have an influence on taking precautions, while actual occurrences of the behavior did not. As suggested by previous research, it may be that an attempt to leave the home is a completely separate phenomenon that causes its own reactions and responses (Butler & Barnett, 1991; Hall, et al., 1995).

In Their Own Words: Caregivers Talk About Attempts at Wandering and Being Lost Inside the Home

"In their own words" contains direct quotes from 13 caregivers who participated in qualitative interviews for Salmons' research. There is no attempt

here to draw hard conclusions from these interview snippets, which occur throughout the chapter. While much of the interview material was about experiences with wandering or getting lost outside the home, several caregivers talked about times when the person with dementia attempted to leave home but was stopped, and about the behavior occurring inside the home.

Attempts at wandering

> There have been times where she would want to go home and be very aggravated with people if they didn't take her. So different times she would get her pocketbook and no jacket or anything and go to the front door and someone would have to try to divert her attention and lots of times she would say, 'Well, I'll go tomorrow.' She would have to redeem herself and make it seem like she was giving in but that she was still going to go because she had to see her mother or whatever.

In the following example of attempts at wandering, the behavior was so severe and upsetting that the caregiver had to move the family to a new residence in an effort to control it.

> If I sat down at night after dinner to read the paper and fall off to sleep, he'd be right out the door! So that's when we sold the house and moved to the condo and I put in a deadbolt. He couldn't get out. He'd get up and try it, oh, a hundred times, but he never got upset about it. He'd just go try the door, he couldn't get out and he'd come back and sit down. They suggested I not change his environment but I couldn't stay with him. I couldn't be with him. If I went into the bathroom, I would turn the shower on and he'd keep going out the door on me.

Lost inside the home

In addition to trying to leave the house, being lost inside the home was a difficult behavior for the caregivers interviewed.

> Sometimes during the night she would bang on the doors and she would get dressed and walk around with her pocketbook at night and she wanted to go home. And if she didn't like what we were saying, she would say, 'I'm going to call the police! I gotta get out of here!' Stuff like that.

Seeing the person with dementia lost inside the home served as an alert for the following caregiver, who registered her mother in the Safe Return program as a result:

> She came up here in October and she would be going out the front door to go to the bathroom. She wouldn't remember where anything was, so that made me think

> how much is she getting lost at home because it seems like whenever she comes to visit and she's in a new environment, it's more of a prelude to what's going to happen to her when she's at home.

On the other hand, findings regarding Salmons' first two hypotheses—that considering wandering to be a problem *was not* associated with using a greater number of precautions, and that caregivers of people who have wandered or gotten lost in the past *did not* use a significantly greater number of precautions, even if they had experienced wandering directly—seem to contradict previous research concerning the general use of safety precautions for this population. While others have found an association between a history of unsafe behavior or accidents and an increased sense of concern or use of safety precautions (Devor, Wang, Renvall, Feigal, & Ramsdell, 1994; Lach, et al., 1995; Russell & Champion, 1996; Watzke & Smith, 1994), Salmons suggests that when wandering is isolated as an individual safety matter—instead of being grouped with other household safety concerns—the effect no longer holds true. In her qualitative interviews, all of the caregivers named a problem other than wandering as being the most critical. Concerns about falling in the house or getting burned on the stove, for example, were at the forefront of their concerns, even if they had experienced wandering in the past. There may be just too many competing issues for caregivers to address, such as getting hurt in the house or the dangerous problem of driving. As Coulton suggests, "when barriers outweigh supports, the problem of failure to engage in preventive behavior may result" (1978, p. 306).

The use of precautions, especially on the behalf of another person, is clearly a complex phenomenon. We reviewed numerous sources related to this phenomenon, including writings on caregivers' use of precautions to prevent wandering; factors associated with general preventive health behavior; and the importance of both safety and independence when responding to and evaluating the risk of wandering.

In Their Own Words: Caregivers Talk About Their Practices and Attitudes Toward Wandering Behavior

Caregiver responses, when asked about wandering and the potential risk, ranged from not having had any experiences and not being concerned at all, to being worried a great deal as a result of a wandering episode. (About 68% of Salmons' larger study sample of 336 caregivers considered wandering to be a problem.)

> I don't worry about wandering. I don't know, maybe I should but she's very content. She stays in her apartment all day. I don't do any day care or anything. I was feeling kind of guilty about that but I've talked with people at [the hospital]. She's content to stay at home. She likes being in that environment. She does the wash or whatever. I just don't have the problem. It just never happened. I don't think it's going to happen. She's 88 years old, she's still very with it, very independent.

> I don't know if she's ever going to wander! She never . . . I leave her in the car. When we go places, sometimes I might just run in real quick and leave her in the car and she stays there. It's just not a problem.

But while wandering was not a concern for some, four of the 13 caregivers indicated that the person with dementia had wandered and been lost outside the home, causing the caregiver to worry about the behavior occurring in the future:

> When the wandering happened, that was such a huge worry that we hadn't thought about before because it had never happened before. We were beside ourselves thinking about what we were going to do. And then, it didn't happen for a few months so you think that was a one-shot deal, it's not going to happen again.

> When I think of her wandering off . . . I mean she could fall and hit her head, she could really hurt herself wandering outside the house. So that is definitely a huge consideration. And like I said, now we're having a little reprieve because the weather's bad and it's cold. But, come the nice weather, I'm sure that will be a consideration again. I'll really have more concerns about her being alone for long periods of time. I'm sure come the spring or summer, I'll have to do something about having her go some place or having more people come in and check her. Because then when it starts happening all the time you have to be with them all the time and then you don't have a life, you can't work, you can't do anything else.

> It's really ironic, I think at one of those (family support group) meetings, but I thought 'I don't have to worry because she's never tried it.' But boy, after that happened, I really . . . that really scared me. I never really had that problem and I never thought she would wander. But what I'm saying is, don't go by what you think because they're going to do something else. You have to be prepared for anything and I wasn't for that, and I am so thankful that nothing happened to her.

> I worry a lot about her going out at night, that's my major worry about it. It worries me more when I think about it, when I talk about it.

Use of Precautions

While research on caregivers' use of precautions for this problem behavior is growing, it is also limited, with most studies reporting on *types* of precautions taken. In a study aimed at identifying modifications made by caregivers to the homes of people with dementia and measuring the effectiveness of each modification, Calkins and Namazi (1991) found that 46 different modifications were made for wandering. The modifications most frequently made included "adding a dead bolt or chain lock, hanging a curtain in front of the door to disguise it, moving a piece of furniture in front of the door to limit access to it, and locking the screen door" (pp. 26–27). These modifications were largely successful: 73% worked well, 18% worked somewhat, and 7% did not work at all.

In a pilot study aimed at determining which safety problems were most common in a study population and exploring the relationship between dementia severity and safety concerns, Lach, Reed, Smith, and Carr (1995) addressed unsafe behavior, accidents and precautions. In this study of 35 community-residing persons with Alzheimer's disease and their caregivers, 25 caregivers (71%) reported that the patients they were caring for engaged in unsafe behavior. "Wandering was the most common safety problem, reported by 37% of the caregivers" (p. 161) and the most common accidents were cuts, falls and getting lost. Sixty-eight percent of the caregivers reported taking precautions to help the person avoid accidents and 54% reported using general supervision. Caregivers were more likely to take safety precautions when dealing with persons with more severe dementia than with those with mild dementia. A history of unsafe behavior or accidents was also associated with the use of precautions.

The authors suggest that "while many caregivers are practicing some form of safety precautions, they may not be aware of all their options or the best way to prevent accidents. For example, wandering was the most common problem, but only one family reported using an identification bracelet" (Lach, et al., 1995, p. 162).

Similarly, in an attempt to understand caregivers' use of precautions, Pynoos, Cohen, and Lucas (1989) suggest that "because of the temporary nature of many behaviors, caregivers may be reluctant to introduce a change or to simplify a task. Instead, the caregiver may provide additional support and attention to the person in order to prevent an accident or to accomplish a specific task. . . . Adjusting the environment may provide the needed support for the person to maintain function and independence" (p. 7). They also suggest that "reluctance to make changes on the part of the caregiver may also come from the negative image of a stigmatized environment, cost of making changes, difficulty in identifying resources or uncertainty over whether the modification will be effective. Yet, many preventative measures are nontherapeutic in appearance, low cost, and relatively simple to make" (p. 7).

In the Salmons study, caregivers of those who have poor vision, are in the late stages of the disease, and have more limitations in their activities of daily living (ADLs), reported using a significantly higher number of precautions.

Finally, summarizing findings on home modifications in general, Gitlin and Corcoran (1996) write:

> The few studies that describe home environments of individuals with dementia suggest that caregivers do implement a range of home modifications. . . . However, enhancement strategies or environmental changes that facilitate functional performance have been found to be underutilized by family caregivers. Additionally, it has been shown that the strategies caregivers implement may need to be refined or modified to maximize their effectiveness (p. 29).

Types of Precautions

Also in the Salmons study, 88% of caregivers reported using at least one of 11 precautions. These included:

1. using night-lights (69%);
2. encouraging movement and exercise in safe areas (58%);
3. playing relaxing music (46%);
4. hiding car keys (30%);
5. placing door locks out of sight, either very high or very low (30%);
6. setting up a safe area in home where s/he can wander at night (26%);
7. using window guards or locks (25%);
8. installing monitor or alarm (22%);
9. putting hedges or fence around yard (14%);
10. using childproof doorknob covers (8%); and
11. disguising doors with curtain or screen (5%).

Precautions 2 through 11 either directly or indirectly address wandering behavior. On the other hand, the most-used precaution—a night-light—is the least likely preventive measure for wandering, although it makes great sense in avoiding other safety problems such as falls. (Caregivers mentioned use of some other precautions, including securing medications, a child safety gate, removing the battery from the car, negotiating with the person with dementia, and using dogs as companions).

Salmons found a number of positive relationships regarding the use of precautions:

- As expected, professional caregivers reported using a significantly higher number of precautions.
- Being limited in activities of daily living was the strongest positive determinant on number of precautions used.

Also using significantly more precautions were:

- Those who cared for someone who had wandered any time;
- Those who cared for someone who had tried to leave home but was stopped in time (The number of attempts to leave home was positively associated with the number of precautions taken.);
- Those who cared for someone who experienced a serious consequence from wandering; and
- Those who had had the police involved a greater number of times.

Contrary to expectations, the use of services in the community, number of services used, and support group membership were not significant predictors of number of precautions taken. And at the other end of the spectrum, using significantly fewer precautions, were:

- Those caring for people with better vision. In fact, having better vision had the greatest negative effect on number of precautions used to prevent or decrease wandering;
- Those who cared for a person with dementia who comes and goes as he or she pleases and/or goes out by him or herself (averaging 3.32 to 4.43 precautions for other caregivers); and
- Older caregivers.

In Their Own Words: Caregivers Talk About Precautions

When asked about precautions taken to decrease or prevent the person with dementia from wandering or getting lost outside the home, caregivers talked specifically about the effectiveness of various strategies, including using locks; relying on neighbors; registering in the Safe Return program and wearing that program's bracelet and other forms of identification; using alarms, bells, or monitors; providing cues; hiding the car keys; and talking and reasoning with the person with dementia.

(Identification was not included in the count of precautions in the Salmons study as it not only represents a postwandering safety precaution, but survey data were drawn from families enrolled in the Alzheimer's Association's national Safe Return program. More than two-thirds of the caregivers reported using identification products, including about 37% who had sewn identification into the person's clothing.)

Using locks

> Even after that, when I'd go to bed and we'd lock all the doors with the key and I felt like a jailer, I had all the keys with me, I still would worry that she would get out. It was awful! We were all locked in tight but I thought, she'd go out the window, I mean, all these crazy thoughts. And I'd check all the windows and we have new windows and they have double locks, and I thought this is terrible.

> Things started to get really bad and that really scared me so we put dead bolts on all the doors.

> Everything you can think of, we tried! Four outside doors all of which we got new deadbolt locks, the keys were always in my possession. The windows were eventually all he could get out of. Then my son fixed them so that they only opened a few inches. And yet if I ever trusted him and left the door inadvertently opened for half an hour to go out and get the mail and forget to lock it again, he'd be gone.

> We put a special lock on the door for safety. Something that fit over the handle. That worked to some degree but when he wants to go, it is amazing! With the precautions—the stop sign on the door and the locks—it was really trial and error, this works, this doesn't.

Relying on neighbors

Five of the 13 caregivers spoke about the importance of neighbors when thinking about and dealing with the risk and experience of wandering:

> The neighbors knew. Everybody in the neighborhood knew. When they saw him, they'd bring him home. I would rarely go out and look for him because I felt I had to stay here and wait for the police or whomever to return him.

> If someone saw him on the first floor going near the door, they would call my mother or they'd say, 'You have to go back upstairs now.' A community thing. We sort of set up this system. She had a friend who had a police radio and the friend would hear when my mother would call to say he was missing so that meant everybody would send the kids out or go out to see if they could find him. As he became worse and his wandering more frequent, everyone kept an eye out for him, particularly if he was in pajamas!

The neighbors would say, 'We saw him!' and we'd go down and find him.

The police also know her. We've lived in this town all our lives. The police know the situation, the neighbors know.

Identification

We had the bracelet on so that he would have it and my mother sewed his name in his clothes and things like that. So if he took the bracelet off, he had something on all his clothes, even his pajamas. He would take the bracelet off. It's like he knew. It was sad, yet it was funny at times. I don't know how he would get it off, if he chewed it off or what, but he would get it off!

Get the ID bracelet. If they won't wear it, keep trying. They're going to reach a point some day when they're not even going to know and she was just about getting there.

Registering in Safe Return made me feel better, in a way. She has the necklace but I'm not sure if she would use it or if she was lost, she would ask for help. She would probably just keep on going, trying to find her way by herself. Unless she passed out or something, you know, no one would come up and look at her necklace! But that's what she wanted, was a necklace. You know, half of me feels like the Alzheimer's thing should be a huge white sticker that you wear on their back so that people know she's in trouble and if she's lost. I'm just not sure if she would ask for help, but then people would take advantage of her or whatever. I know that you can't do that but something that's more obvious, that sticks out.

Alarms, bells, monitors

We tried putting bells, she'd come and take them down. I have a couple of cowbells and I hung them on the doors, I put one on her bedroom door and she didn't like that so she would constantly take that off.

I have a monitor in my bedroom because our bedroom is quite a distance.

Providing cues

When I'm out, I write down where I'm going and all the details. When I send him out, for example to buy stamps at the post office, I give him an envelope to bring the stamps back in. When I ask him to go to [the pharmacy], I give him the empty box of whatever I want him to buy. These are cues for him that keep him on track.

I call her twice a day. I check in on her no matter what time I come in at night. I check in on her. . . . If she's sleeping, that means good news. That means that she's had a good night before sleeping.

When we finally had him diagnosed, we worked with a visiting nurse to try to do things like put signs at the doors in big letters 'STOP,' which didn't work.

Hiding the car keys

I had hidden the car keys but he found them. We are getting rid of the car after Thanksgiving. Our family needs to use it over the holidays but after that, we are going to get rid of it. He sometimes drives me places. He's an excellent driver.

Talking and reasoning

We talk to her a lot about whenever she wanted to go for a walk to tell somebody and if nobody was here to wait for somebody to come back. We would always take her for a walk.

In the last year, he lost touch with all reality, so trying to explain didn't make any sense. We'd explain, but because he couldn't hold on to what we said, 'Don't go out of the house' did not work. We would try to convince him logically why he shouldn't do it, which didn't work.

I'll say, 'Mom, if you get out of bed in the middle of the night, and come to the back door and it's totally dark, you know that everybody's sleeping.' I've convinced her to stay in bed—well, I haven't really convinced her, but most of the time, when it's time to get up, I will go over and wake her up. So, I'll say to her, 'You just stay in bed and when I wake up, I'll come get you.' And she'll say, 'You know, that's really good advice,' and then she'll look at me and laugh and say, 'but I'll probably forget.'

Altering living arrangements

Throughout the qualitative interviews, there was sufficient concern for the safety of the person with dementia to cause relocation to the caregiver's residence.

My mom lived alone in her apartment in New York City until last November when I took her to live with me. I had known for at least 5 years that she shouldn't be living alone. I didn't really know why, I didn't know that she has Alzheimer's or whatever it is she has. My sister, who lives in New York, was really close to her and neither of them would admit there was a problem.

We talked to her for about a year about coming and staying with us, with my husband and I, and she didn't want to leave [her hometown], and 'No, no, I'm fine, I can do it myself!' But things were just starting to slide down and getting worse, as far as I was concerned and I was very worried. My sister, saying, 'Oh,

> let her stay. She'll be fine. When something really happens, then you'll have to make a decision.' But one time we talked to her, and she really should not have been alone, many of her neighbors had said that to us. But she didn't want to leave her house. But there's a time, I think, when you have to kind of step in a little bit. So anyway, she did agree to come and stay with us. She wanted to stay in her home, we looked at assisted housing, but she wouldn't have any part of that, we looked at senior housing, she didn't want that. So we kept her in her house and she did better than we thought but she was still confused. She was there for 2 years.
>
> And I always think that I took my mother, I took her out of her environment, her little safety with her house and I brought her here because I thought it was the best thing—things like that. And I think anybody, if they feel, try anything you can to keep them at home, which I think we did, but she was failing.
>
> It's hard, you can't just take somebody and make them. How can you do that? One of the neighbors said, 'Well, I don't think you can make somebody go with you,' but we tried to convince her to come. But my god, when their safety is an issue, then you've got to do something. I couldn't stand by and watch that! We finally convinced her to come and live with us.

One additional, major modification, providing 24-hour supervision, is often recommended by many experts as the most effective precaution for protecting people with dementia against unsafe wandering, but is also a difficult one for caregivers to implement and manage, both practically and personally.

In the Salmons study, caregivers spoke of the difficulties associated with providing 24-hour supervision, and about the struggles involved with deciding living arrangements, especially if the person with dementia was living on his or her own. They also talked about the need to take care of their own families and households, the social isolation that can occur as a result of always being in the caregiving role, and the struggle with concerns for both the safety and the independence of the person with dementia in their care.

24-Hour Supervision

Caregiver characteristics

Salmons found four of seven caregiver characteristics significantly associated with the 24-hour supervision. Caregivers' age, relationship, health status, and employment status were all significant. Caregivers who were older, spouses of the persons with dementia, or not employed were more likely than other groups to provide 24-hour supervision. With regard to caregiver health, those who reported themselves to be in fair health were more likely than other caregivers to be providing around-the-clock supervision.

Characteristics of person with dementia

The age, gender, or race of the person with dementia was not significantly associated with 24-hour supervision. However, both marital status and living arrangement were significant. The odds of receiving 24-hour supervision were three times greater for those who were married.

Use of community services

Caregivers who had been members of dementia family support groups were significantly more likely to provide 24-hour supervision. Odds of providing 24-hour supervision increased almost two and a half times if the caregiver was a member of a dementia family support group.

Experience With Wandering Behavior

Caregivers of those who have usually wandered in the afternoon were more likely than others to offer around-the-clock supervision. Among those caring for someone who had wandered or been lost in the past, about 60% reported providing 24-hour supervision.

Reflecting on the findings regarding numbers of precautions taken, those with dementia who communicate well were 40% less likely to be supervised 24 hours a day. Also, as was expected, those who come and go as they please and/or go out by themselves were 75% less likely to receive 24-hour supervision. And those who live alone were 85% less likely to receive around-the-clock supervision.

In Their Own Words: Caregivers Talk About 24-Hour Supervision

Asked about the amount of supervision provided for the person with dementia, caregivers in the qualitative interviews offered mixed reactions. Some talked about the struggle of knowing 24-hour supervision is necessary but not being able to practically provide it, some spoke about providing 24-hour supervision and the difficulties it presents, and some talked about being supportive and comfortable with the person with dementia spending time alone, even if they had wandered or been lost in the past.

> With my own family, I couldn't stay with them 24 hours. But it was getting to the point that something had to be done or somebody was going to get hurt.

> He can't leave her at all now. He'll walk down the 100 yards to the little general store and the post office but other than that he takes her on all his errands in the car. He doesn't really let her out of his sight anymore. He doesn't even go to the barber anymore. He's bought himself a clipper, an electric clipper and my mother cuts his hair now! Number one, it means that he's not getting out and interacting with anybody else. He's coping, too, so he doesn't have to leave her alone.

> He does go out alone. I both allow it and encourage it.

> Yes, of course, he can go out alone. I feel confident that he's okay if I tell him where he's going and if he's not gone for very long. I get more anxious if he's gone for a long time. He stays by himself. Today, I was out from 9 a.m. to 4 p.m.

Preventive Health Behavior

While the previous section reviewed writings specifically on caregivers' use of precautions for wandering, the literature concerning general preventive health behavior, especially that which is done on behalf of a dependent person such as a cognitively-impaired adult, is also important to consider.

Preventive health behavior is a complex phenomenon. In an attempt to understand the complexities involved in taking preventive actions for other people, a conceptual model by Ohta and Ohta (1990) adapted by Silverstein, Hyde, and Ohta (1993, p. 97) identified four factors as being important to dementia caregivers when they decide whether to implement home adaptation recommendations for those with cognitive impairments:

1. the likelihood that a particular problem will occur without the adaptation;
2. the severity of that problem;
3. the potential effectiveness of the adaptation; and
4. the cost of the adaptation.

Guided by this framework, Silverstein and colleagues found that "while caregivers perceived certain target problems to be very serious, they did not perceive their family members as susceptible" (1993, p. 104). They also added an interesting point, that "the variability of behaviors over the course of the disease may make it difficult for caregivers to assess their family member's personal degree of susceptibility" (p. 104). This issue of personal susceptibility has also been found to be a factor in other studies investigating the use of protective strategies (Collins, 1996).

Safety vs. Independence

In addition to factors associated with preventive health behavior, the literature also addresses the issues of safety and autonomy which are often involved when dealing with dementia and problems such as wandering (Collopy, 1995; Haley & Coleton, 1992; Hirschfeld, 1985; Hofland, 1994; Kapp, 1995; Kelly, 1994; Roberto, 1994; Taft, Delaney, Seman, & Stansell, 1993).

While much of this literature is based in ethics, its content offers important insight into the intricacies of the caregiver's decision-making process. For that reason, and because the struggle between the two ideals—safety and autonomy—is of such importance to people with dementing illnesses and to all those involved in their care, we will take some time here to examine these issues.

Many have written about the safety side of the debate, often noting the importance of a diminished decision-making capacity for the person with dementia. Collopy (1995), for example, writes about the conflicts between independence and safety and the complications introduced by the question of mental capacity, suggesting that in conflicts of this sort:

> The individual must be able to understand the consequences of choice and behavior, to grasp the relationship between means and goals, and to appreciate potential risks and benefits. Ultimately, he or she must be able to assume the burdens as well as the benefits of independence—in short, to calculate the darker aspects of choice and to take responsibility for the harms that independence can bring (p. 47).

More specifically, McGlynn and Schacter (1989) cite the fact that "most dementias are accompanied by *anosognosia*, which is failure to recognize one's own cognitive deficits" (p. 144). They contend that "a corollary to this is that frustration, irritability, and agitation almost invariably accompany any reminder to the patient that a problem exists" (p. 144). Flaherty and Raia (1994) agree, suggesting that "typically, people with Alzheimer's are unaware of their deficits or incapacities, and if they are aware, will minimize them" (p. 88).

Along the same lines, Noyes and Silva (1993) write about the influence of paternalism in justifying locked special care units for people with dementia. Such a justification is based on the theory that many people with dementia have a limited capacity to choose right from wrong and therefore, have a limited degree of autonomy. While their writings include the opposite view concerning the importance of independence, Noyes' and Silva's views on wandering, specifically, suggest that wandering behaviors "can rarely be considered autonomous actions since they lack the characteristics of intentionality, understanding, and voluntariness" (p. 13). They suggest that "the harms prevented from occurring or the benefits provided to the person outweigh the loss of independence and the sense of invasion caused by the interference; the person's condition seriously limits his or her ability to choose autonomously" (p. 14).

Lipscomb (1988) also emphasizes the safety dimension in the safety versus independence debate by writing that "deflection and dissimilation no longer are useful when dementia becomes full-blown, and the caregiver must assume the role of benevolent parent to prevent the patient from harm, wandering, and uncontrolled aggression" (p. 29).

But while many have written about the importance of safety when dealing with wandering behavior, the competing theme of independence and autonomy must be considered when trying to understand what influences caregivers' use of precautions.

Collopy (1995) highlights the struggles between the two ideals, noting that "in both institutional and community-based care, conflicts between safety of the frail elderly and their independence are very often resolved in favor of safety" (p. 44), but making the important point that "safety is not an absolute value. It stands within the context of other values, and this context varies with the elderly individual—the one who must ultimately bear loss of independence or greater risks to safety" (p. 46).

And Epstein (1994) reminds us that "while wandering is a common symptom of Alzheimer's disease or related dementia, providers should not assume that all residents with dementia lack decision-making capacity" (p. 42).

An example of a formal response to this debate is cited by Flaherty and Raia (1994). They reference a handout accompanying training materials for Massachusetts Elder Protective and Elder-at-Risk caseworkers titled, "A Theory of Adult Protection," which offers this guidance:

> When interests compete, the adult client is the only person you are charged to serve; not the community concerned about the safety, the landlords concerned about property, citizens concerned about crime or mortality, or families concerned about their own health or finances.

> When interests compete, the adult client is in charge of decision-making until she/he delegates responsibility voluntarily to another or the court grants responsibility to another.
>
> Freedom is more important than safety; that is, the person can choose to live in harm or even self-destructively provided she/he is competent to choose, does not harm others, and commits no crimes (pp. 82–83).

Flaherty and Raia felt this generally well-intentioned advice was inappropriate when applied to clients in all but the earlier stages of a progressive dementing illness. What is interesting to note, in that regard, is that other research suggests caregivers may be more sensitive to concerns for autonomy than the elders they care for (Horowitz, Silverstone, & Reinhardt, 1991). In a study designed to examine possible conflicts with personal autonomy in family caregiving relationships, the authors found that, "Caregivers seemed more sensitive to the needs of the (memory-impaired) older person, even if they were perceived as harmful, and were more open to negotiating a compromise that respected these needs" (p. 28). In fact, the elder care recipients in the study "were primarily concerned with ensuring the health and safety of the older people in the vignettes, and saw these concerns as overriding questions of self-determination or personal choice" (p. 26).

Of those in the Salmons study who had wandered or been lost in the past, one-fourth reported that the person with dementia comes and goes as he or she pleases and/or goes out by him or herself. When asked directly about supervision, 40% of the caregivers reported that the person with dementia was not supervised the entire day and night. Even when caregivers indicated that wandering had occurred and that they may be concerned about it, many with dementia in their care still go out alone or are left unsupervised.

These findings agree with research regarding driving (see chapter 3) conducted by Pynoos and colleagues, which found that "although half of the caregivers of the AD patients who currently drove expressed concerns, only 13% felt the patient should discontinue driving. . . . Many families are unwilling or unable to take the right to drive away from the Alzheimer's patient" (1989, p. 8).

In Their Own Words: Caregivers Talk About Safety Versus Independence

The struggle between encouraging a person's safety and preserving his or her independence and autonomy emerged as a central theme in our qualitative interviews with caregivers. For some, the diminished decision-making capacity of the person in their care influenced their own decision-making about safety and personal autonomy.

> Sometimes you catch yourself and remember that she doesn't have that ability to plan, to use judgment.

And in the first example below, the caregiver portrays the difficulties involved and the ambivalence felt when trying to evaluate the relative importance of safety risks and quality of life:

> I was talking with them (siblings) about what would be one of the symptoms or what would be one of the things that would make us realize that it would be time for her (mother) to go to assisted living and I think that her getting lost would be one of the signs that she'd be ready. But I guess the question would be whether she's lost or not. My brother thought that might be jumping the gun, let's really wait and see. My sister goes back and forth on that, she really thinks that her quality of life right now is much better than she would have it anywhere else and she wants to keep her where she is and she is willing to take the risk. She's willing to gamble with it more than I might be willing to. My sister is adamant about having her stay there, because she's lived in that house for 35 years or something like that.

Similarly, the following caregiver statement highlights the struggle felt when faced with a threat to the person's safety and a threat to his or her quality of life.

> And once that happened, then it was like if she was going to do that, what were we ever going to do? We couldn't lock her in the house, how can you lock someone in the house on a beautiful summer day? I could tell my kids to go to bed and they would go. My mother can say no and there's nothing you can do.

In addition to being concerned about safety and quality of life, several of the caregivers indicated the importance of protecting the reputation of the person in their care:

> We finally found our way back but we kind of kept it between ourselves because it was almost like it was important to him not to let anyone know. You know, that he couldn't find his way home. So I never told anyone.

> I want to talk to him still. I don't want him to feel . . . I don't want to treat that guy with kid-gloves. I just don't. I want him to feel like he's my equal and I'm

> going to treat him like he was my pal, like before all this happened. But it is tough, it is tough. The guy was always on the top of his game.

A further difficulty associated with the issue of autonomy is the threat to the dignity of the person with dementia, and the caregivers' efforts to preserve it.

> So we're trying to always think of things to do that wouldn't—I didn't want to embarrass her or, you know, that's terrible. You think of everything you do and it's . . . you're taking away their dignity.

> It's kind of hard to think that this is the man I'm married to for 52 years and he's not the same. You have to treat him almost like a baby.

> It's just like taking care of an infant. But she's grateful for the care and I'm respecting who she is. Alzheimer's doesn't take away everything. So much has been stripped away, she's lost so much else, she's lost so much of the cover, it's almost as if she's exposed her essence a lot of times.

A Review of the General Findings on Caregiver Response to Wandering Behavior

In order to improve the effectiveness of interventions for wandering and getting lost outside the home and to promote prevention of this behavior, it is necessary to predict what circumstances or strategies are likely to increase success. To begin to answer these questions, it is essential to first understand what factors influence or determine preventative behavior for this problem. The foregoing section of chapter 4 begins, we hope, to build such an understanding. The suggestions below reiterate or follow from the results and themes discussed in the previous pages pertinent to caregivers' current responses to wandering behavior and use of specific precautions.

Summary

While the collective findings discussed above suggest that many of these caregivers were aware of the risks associated with wandering and had experienced its problems firsthand, not everyone regarded this behavior as a serious problem, with Salmons' research showing that only 68% of the caregivers who had experienced wandering considered it to be a problem.

There are several possible explanations for the discrepancy between the proportion of caregivers who have experienced the person with dementia wandering or getting lost outside the home and those for whom it was described as a problem. Salmons' qualitative interviews suggest that this disease is accompanied by a myriad of problems. Caregivers may be dealing with other things that are more pressing. Perhaps problems like incontinence and forgetting to eat or bathe, which occur throughout the day, nearly every day, are more problematic than a behavior such as wandering, which may be more intermittent.

When considering the body of literature, the data support the notion that caregivers do learn from experience. More specifically, their preventive actions seem to be influenced not by direct exposure to wandering incidents, but by a myriad of experiences with the behavior. As noted earlier, a long history of research showing that preventive health behavior, especially that which is done on behalf of a dependent person such as a cognitively impaired adult, is a complex phenomenon, and may help explain these results.

Caregivers talked about their feelings of personal susceptibility (e.g., "I just don't have the problem. It just never happened. I don't think it's going to happen," and, "I never really had a problem with it and I never thought she would wander."), quotes which seem to concur with Coulton's suggestion regarding beliefs about severe impact. More than a third of the caregivers in our survey who had experienced wandering did not consider it to be a problem.

Salmons' qualitative material also related to another of Coulton's points concerning beliefs about the effectiveness of preventive actions. Many of the caregivers talked about the difficulty involved in finding precautions that worked well. They reported problems in using all types of precautions. Several caregivers complained about the practical utility of an identification bracelet.

When considering sociocultural factors, Coulton (1978) writes that "Norms, sanctions, or collectively held beliefs of groups to which an individual belongs may affect his beliefs in these areas"—beliefs about the etiology of the illness, severity of illness, and how illness can be prevented (p. 300). Such groups include families, neighbors, peers, work groups, socioeconomic groups, and ethnic groups. Indeed, family members and neighbors do seem to have an impact. In several cases cited in our interviews, decisions surrounding the use of precautions for wandering, living alone, and driving were determined by several members of the family rather than the caregiver alone. Neighbors also played a part. Many caregivers reported that neighbors helped in finding the person with dementia who had wandered and was lost. In addition, for people with dementia living alone, neighbors often alerted caregivers to problems they had observed in the caregivers' absence.

In addition to the ideas discussed above, it is also likely that the psychological readiness of the caregiver has an impact on the use of precautions against wandering. In studies of compliance with social and safety recommendations, researchers found failure to accept a diagnosis and the need for treatment to be the most common reason for noncompliance (Devor, Wang, Renvall, Feigal, & Ramsdell, 1994). Both our quantitative and qualitative results support this idea. For example, those who were diagnosed more recently tended to use fewer precautions and were less likely to provide 24-hour supervision. Just as it is common for caregivers to tend to deny the presence of the disease and its symptoms at the beginning of the disease process, it may also be likely that they deny the need for precautions, even though a behavior such as wandering is occurring. Chenoweth and Spencer concur, suggesting that "Families had difficulty understanding that a person eventually would not be able to read or write, or that wandering, lack of manners, or constant pacing could be part of the disease . . . with few exceptions, families were astonished when they recognized the extent of impairment in thought, judgment, and reasoning" (1986, p. 269).

As evidenced by ours and others' research, any attempt to understand influences on caregivers' use of precautions to prevent a person with dementia from wandering outside the home must consider the family's values and beliefs concerning the independence, autonomy, and capacity of that person (Hofland, 1994; Roberto, 1994). The qualitative interviews highlighted the fact that caregivers often struggle with concerns for the person's safety while also worrying about the person's degree of independent living, quality of life, and sense of dignity. In fact, some wandering precautions (e.g., hiring someone to take walks with the person with dementia) were seen by caregivers as enhancing both safety and quality of life simultaneously. Additionally, the work of Becker and Maiman (1975), and Devor and colleagues (1994) suggests that "Measures that require personal or financial sacrifice or which disrupt well-established habits or a family unit will not be followed unless the benefit is perceived to outweigh the sacrifice" (p. M172).

The importance of both personal freedom and safety came through not only when talking about wandering and precautions used, but also when discussing the issues of living alone and driving. Efforts to respect the wishes of the person with dementia and safeguard against various hazards is especially difficult in the early stages of a dementing illness, when lapses of memory are occasional, and autonomy may still be a relevant concept (Hofland, 1994).

Finally, in trying to understand preventive behavior for adults who are cognitively impaired, it is important to consider the influence of the person with the impairment. Quotes from caregiver interviews illustrate this point on several levels (e.g., "I could tell my kids to go to bed and they would go. My mother can say no and there's nothing you can do," and, "He would take the [ID] bracelet off. It's like he knew. I don't know how he would get it off, if he chewed it off or what, but he would get it off!"). Lach and colleagues found, similarly, that "One of the barriers to using precautions is resistance by the patient. Caregivers may give up on the precautions to avoid arguments or catastrophic reactions" (1995, p. 162).

In summary, the theoretical implications of all the data discussed here lead us to stress the importance of certain attitudes and influences which affect caregivers in their preventive behaviors:

- Concerns about issues of safety as well as with preserving the independence of the person with dementia.
- Feelings of personal susceptibility to the risks posed by wandering behavior.
- Perceived costs of and barriers to taking precautionary measures.
- Perceptions concerning the effectiveness of various precautions.
- The influence of family members—decisions around issues of risk and prevention are rarely made by the primary caregiver alone.
- Finally, a most important piece—the influence of the person with dementia.

Until now, the likelihood that caregivers have recognized wandering and becoming lost as a high-risk behavior and have identified appropriate strategies to minimize harmful consequences of that behavior has been minimal—hit or miss at best. While many of the coping strategies have grown out of the tried-and-true category of caregiver experience and should be shared with others, other strategies may actually be detrimental in the long run. Basically, caregivers who have not yet experienced catastrophic consequences from a wandering episode have been nothing less than lucky. This chapter has illustrated both through quantitative research findings and qualitative anecdotal accounts how caregivers currently respond to wandering behavior. In the next chapter, we will explore the response of law enforcement to individuals with dementing illnesses who wander from their homes and become lost.

CHAPTER 5

Law Enforcement and Technology

There is a significant chance that police officers will be asked to respond to reports of older people who are missing from their homes or from care facilities. Most officers, at some point, will come in contact with an elderly person out on the street, lost and confused (Flaherty & Scheft, 1995). Rowe and Glover (2001) found that less than 4% of memory-impaired adults who wander away from home are able to return unassisted. And as noted in the introduction and in chapter 2, Koester (2001), using data also cited in this book, estimates that more than 127,000 critical wandering incidents involving people with dementia occur each year. His estimate is startling. More startling, given the Alzheimer's Association's estimates of prevalence rates for the disease and the aging of the baby-boomer generation, is that Koester also predicts that by the year 2040, this number could grow to more than a half million cases.

Police officers may also become involved in cases where neglect of a memory impaired elder is a precipitating cause of a wandering incident. It is worth repeating here, as we said in the Introduction to Part II, that current responses to wandering behavior, across the board, are far more crisis-oriented than preventive, including those by law enforcement or related agencies such as search and rescue organizations, or even by manufacturers of safety and alarm devices. Local police may be continually recovering the lost person with dementia and bringing him or her home without any referral to the formal elder service network which, for its part, may be ignoring the full extent of the risk even when such a referral is made. This collective, cursory response may enable the wanderer to continue a high-risk behavior.

Increased media attention to the medical, economic, and social effects of Alzheimer's disease, together with specific education and outreach efforts of agencies such as the national Alzheimer's Association, through its Safe Return Program, have helped draw police attention to this endemic behavior. But in a personal story of the search for her missing mother, Caldwell (1995) explains potential problems with law enforcement and reinforces the need for the training of police:

> My own experience alerts me to the difficulties in working with small police departments. It is often difficult to obtain verification of information entered into police reports. The smaller police agencies in villages and rural towns may be restricted by limited financial resources. Training for officers may be minimal and their knowledge of what to do when an individual vanishes is frequently limited (Caldwell, 1995, pp. 51–52).

And our experience tells us that in urban areas as well, the importance of responding quickly to reports of missing elders, particularly when the elder's memory impairment is not clearly stated, may be overshadowed by the more obvious, and traditional, role of police in responding immediately to reports of criminal activity or medical emergencies.

Of all the programs in effect nationally to address wandering behavior which we investigated, the previously mentioned Safe Return program comes closest to providing a large scale, uniform, proactive, and inexpensive response to wandering incidents. This is not to downplay the good work of other agencies or businesses with the same aims. As the technology of electronic personal locator devices becomes more sophisticated and less expensive (more on this later), all will certainly be able to offer proactive strategies, based on improvements in the miniaturization and accuracy of these devices, to find missing Alzheimer's patients more quickly and with less strain on resources.

The Alzheimer's Association's National Safe Return Program

> It's really ironic. I had information on the ID bracelet, I think at one of those (family support group) meetings, but I thought, "I don't have to worry because she's never tried it, she never wandered. But boy, after that happened, I really . . . that really scared me. So I sent away for the stuff."

> I never really had that problem and I never thought she would wander. But what I'm saying is, don't go by what you think because they're going to do something else. You have to be prepared for anything and I wasn't for that and I am so thankful that nothing happened to her. Get the ID bracelet.

> The police had to bring him home and he said, "He should have a bracelet," and I said, "Well, he knows his name." And the policeman said, "But he doesn't know his address."

The Safe Return program was legislated by Congress in 1992 in an effort to address the individual protection problems associated with wandering behavior in Alzheimer's disease. It is a proactive program designed to safely return missing persons with Alzheimer's disease and related disorders and to train police, emergency personnel and others to recognize the dangers associated with wandering behavior and deal appropriately with them.

The Alzheimer's Association operates Safe Return as a 24-hour national database identification program 365 days a year, with principal funding through the U.S. Justice Department. For a one-time fee, people with Alzheimer's disease or a related disorder are registered for life in the program. (As of this writing the fee is $40, which helps defray the cost of processing registrations and purchasing identification products. It can be waived if necessary, and some states subsidize the cost of registration for eligible residents.)

The Alzheimer's Association operates the central Safe Return registry nationwide through the toll-free Safe Return emergency number, 800-572-1122. All reports of a lost patient, at any time of day or night, are made to the 800-572-1122 number. The Safe Return program is in place throughout the Alzheimer's Association's chapter network in every state, serves registrants and nonregistrants alike, and is readily available to law enforcement agencies responding to lost patient cases. Anyone can call the 800 number with information on a missing or found patient, or to initiate the registration process for a family member or client with a dementing illness.

The vast majority of registrations are filled out for the patient by a family or professional caregiver, who is encouraged to include a recent photograph of the registrant, which can be faxed to police when necessary. Information from the registration form entered into the Safe Return database includes name, address, phone, date of birth, age; personal characteristics such as gender, height, weight, eye color, hair color, race, complexion, and language spoken; any distinguishing features, typical clothing and appearance; any problem behaviors or major medical conditions and medications; caregiver information listing a primary contact person and two other backup contacts; and information listing law enforcement and hospital contacts closest to the registrant's home.

Identification products and educational materials are generally mailed to the primary caregiver. ID products include a bracelet, necklace, key chain, lapel pin, clothing labels, wallet card, and refrigerator magnet. The jewelry and wallet ID are also available to caregivers (for a small added fee, currently

$5). The caregiver IDs are designed to alert others, in the event a primary family caregiver becomes incapacitated, that there is a need to look after the person at home with Alzheimer's. Caregiver IDs can also encourage an otherwise reluctant Alzheimer's patient to wear his or her identification.

Of the various patient ID products, the most commonly used is the Safe Return bracelet (86% in Silverstein & Salmons, 1996). Registrants and caregivers have three choices as to the outward appearance of the bracelet: one has the words "Alzheimer's Association, Safe Return Program" (most commonly chosen), one has only the words "Safe Return," and one has only the Alzheimer's Association's logo with no wording. The backs of all bracelets contain the same information: the patient/registrants' first name, a unique code number, the words "Memory-impaired," and the instruction "To help (first name) call 1-800-572-1122," the program's toll-free emergency number.

All Safe Return 800 number operators are professionals with crisis counseling experience who coordinate efforts to recover Alzheimer's patients who have wandered from a home or facility and become lost. When advised of an Alzheimer's patient who is missing or found wandering, they work with callers, caregivers and police to gather pertinent information to resolve the case quickly and safely. Many local Alzheimer's Association chapters have protocols for after-hours notification of staff in the more complicated cases, and some are also connected to a sophisticated 24-hour fax network which can broadcast alerts to agencies such as police departments and hospitals in targeted communities. All local chapters offer follow-up counseling and service referrals to address the situation which led to the wandering incident.

The Safe Return program recommends that the following four steps be taken immediately when a memory impaired person wanders off:

1. Quickly search the immediate vicinity;
2. Notify local police;
3. Call the Safe Return 800-572-1122 emergency number; and
4. Have someone familiar with the missing patient stay by the phone to assist in the case (and, if possible, call a relative or friend to join you for support).

As of this writing, almost 90,000 people with Alzheimer's disease or a related disorder will have been registered nationally, and 97% of the roughly 7,000 registrants who were reported to Safe Return because they had wandered had been recovered (Alzheimer's Association, 2002).

Research on Safe Return

Evaluations of the Safe Return program have been conducted by various entities, including local Alzheimer's Association chapters. The chapter in St.

Louis surveyed a random sample of its Safe Return registrants (Alzheimer's Association, St. Louis Chapter, 1995) and reported that most respondents (53%) learned about Safe Return through Alzheimer's Association literature or staff; 20% from a doctor or health care provider; 20% from a friend or relative; and 6% from items in the news media. The St. Louis study also found that most caregivers were prompted to enroll patients in the program for preventive reasons, including: fear of wandering and safety reasons (41%); receiving a diagnosis of Alzheimer's or a related dementia (29%); because the person had gotten lost (22%); or because someone suggested enrollment (4%). And while 49% indicated that wandering incidents had occurred before enrollment in the program, a notable 74% indicated there were no wandering incidents since enrollment. Ninety percent reported that they had not called the 800 Safe Return emergency number, and 57% that they had not advised their local police department that they were caring for someone with Alzheimer's. It should also be noted that while roughly two-thirds reported that the ID jewelry was being worn as was intended, another third reported that it was not being worn at all.

Similarly, Silverstein and Salmons (1996), in a study conducted with the Massachusetts chapter through the University of Massachusetts Gerontology Institute in Boston, found that 30% of caregivers learned about Safe Return through literature from the Alzheimer's Association; 24% from a doctor or other health care provider; 15% by attending an Alzheimer's family support group; 13% from a friend or relative; and 4% from items in the news media. Registering someone in the Safe Return program was also primarily a preventive measure for caregivers, with 51% reporting that they registered the person because they were concerned about his or her wandering and getting lost in the future (interestingly, 17% of patients experienced their first wandering incident after being registered); and 35% because there had already been a wandering incident.

Echoing the St. Louis study, the UMass study found that 21% of caregivers reported that the registrant did not wear any identification. Of the other 79% who did report ID use in the UMass study, the bracelet, as mentioned, was the most common type (86%). There was a second similar finding: While 239 people enrolled by the Massachusetts chapter had wandered and become lost only 10% of their caregivers reported in the study that they had called the Safe Return 800 emergency number directly in response to a wandering incident. (It is not known how many of these wanderers were registered in Safe Return at the time they wandered.)

Working in conjunction with the Alzheimer's Association's nationwide network of chapters, the Safe Return program trains police, firefighters, paramedics, 911 dispatchers, doctors, nurses, home health care workers, and any others who might, in their professions, encounter a person who has wandered. Properly trained personnel save time and resources by avoiding unnecessary arrests and processing which would allow police more time to spend on patrol.

These trainings also promote more timely and dignified recovery of wanderers which, in turn, lowers the rate of medical intervention needed to treat effects of prolonged exposure to the elements, malnutrition, and injury. Safe Return is involved throughout the search and stays in contact afterward to help prevent future wandering.

The Safe Return program also enjoys support in the form of cooperative arrangements with various state governmental offices across the country. In Massachusetts, for example, the Executive Office of Elder Affairs, which funds a system of community-based elder home care provider agencies serving the greatest number of elder clients in the state, covers the one-time cost of registration in Safe Return. There is also funding for programs providing safety devices for elders who qualify financially, which is available through the federal/state Medicaid program (under the Personal Emergency Response System provision) and through some grants made by local Area Agencies on Aging.

As with the programs outlined below, Safe Return is not a complete answer to wandering behavior. With about 2% of the country's dementia population enrolled, families, agencies, and facilities are not currently taking good advantage of it. Nor are the police. Safe Return logs roughly 2,000 or more cases a year, while there are an estimated 34,000 cases, as noted earlier, which are reported to police each year.

Some Other Examples of Community Law Enforcement Programs in Response to Wandering Behavior

Alzheimer safety books or registries

These are perhaps the most common types of programs offered by police nationwide. Some operate in conjunction with the Alzheimer's Association's national Safe Return program and link dementia wanderers and their caregivers to referral networks; others do not. Local departments compile these registration files primarily to help identify people with Alzheimer's and other memory disorders in situations which call for police assistance. Some safety registries are computerized, some are simply photo albums, and most have some medical information. While these types of programs represent a common police response, many, if not most, departments do not establish them. In those that do, the registries are usually very small (in comparison both with the local community's dementia population and to prevalence estimates of wandering episodes in that population). One likely reason for the lack of registrants is that all information must be supplied voluntarily by caregivers (or staff at facilities such as nursing homes, with caregiver approval) who need to travel to the local police department to register the person with dementia. Given the constant demands of dementia care and the apprehension caregivers may feel about visiting a police station, the paucity of registrants is not surprising. Additionally, demands on officers' time mean that these registries may not always be kept up-to-date. Their effectiveness also depends heavily on officers' awareness of the existence and location of the registry at the police station, its 24-hour availability, and in cases where a memory-impaired person is found wandering in another jurisdiction, on whether the hometown police are ever notified.

There are other, broader police-sponsored registry programs in the community, such as the "File of Life" (in some towns called the "Vial of Life") program, through which a sticker is placed in a conspicuous location—an entryway, for example—alerting first responders such as EMTs that there is a vial attached to the kitchen refrigerator by a magnet which contains general health, medical, and family contact information on the elder.

Project Lifesaver

The Project Lifesaver uses technology consisting of a small transmitter attached to the wrist of an Alzheimer's patient and a receiver that tracks a signal transmitted from this wristlet over radio frequencies. It is in use by search groups in several states, in some areas in conjunction with the Alzheimer's Association's Safe Return program. It is relatively expensive (current estimated cost is over $2,000 for the receiver and about $300 for the transmitter, with a small monthly maintenance charge). This technology may perform better when the receiving equipment is operated by a central law enforcement or search and rescue agency.

Fingerprinting programs

These are less common than local safety registries as a response to dementia wandering, but some police departments do offer free fingerprinting programs. Their effectiveness would seem to be limited to identifying dementia wanderers who are found but cannot communicate, who have not been reported to the police as missing, and who have no ID with them. This type of program is more likely to be used for children than for people with dementia.

Video ID programs

These are even less common, but some local police departments will make a free, very short videotape to help with the retrieval of missing children, or adults with Alzheimer's disease. The video ID shows physical size, manner of speaking, and other individual traits. Caregiver use and program effectiveness depend on issues very similar to those applying to local safety registries. Again, this type of program is more likely to be used for children than for people with dementia.

Educational materials for caregivers

Some police departments offer educational brochures for caregivers. One example of such a police-sponsored initiative occurred in Raleigh, North Carolina, in response to police generated data indicating that 10% of missing-person calls in 1997 involved confused elderly people. The Raleigh brochure, "Missing Persons: A Guide for Caregivers of the Elderly," contains information on how to prevent wandering, and steps which can make it easier for police to find dementia wanderers.

Wandering Technology Devices and Resource Information

That caregivers want more immediate solutions than those categorized above is apparent not only in interviews with caregivers but also in media interest in emerging personal locator technology around the world, as evidenced in this 1999 report filed by Associated Press reporter Daniel Woolls from Madrid, Spain:

> The death of an Alzheimer's patient who strayed from home and tumbled down a hillside has prompted an ambitious project to use satellites to find victims of the disease if they become lost. The idea, developed by a Spanish Alzheimer's association and due to be introduced late this year, is to have patients wear a tracer that would activate if the user goes beyond a set radius from home. The device would emit a signal that bounces off a satellite and into a monitoring center where staff would call relatives and determine if the patient is in fact missing. If so, police are given real-time coordinates mapped by the satellite and sent out to find the patient.

While the programs listed above illustrate a range of precautions taken by law enforcement to counteract wandering behavior, most relevant to this discussion in this chapter is the body of research on the use of technology to respond to the behavior. A brief review of the literature on this technology follows, and is organized around three main themes: first, an overall description of wanderer control technology currently available; second, research concerning the likely demand for such systems by caregivers in the community; and, third, possible barriers and advantages to using these technological interventions.

It is helpful to know that while the systems vary with respect to technical features, capabilities, and available options, in general there are three types. One is a relatively simple boundary-crossing alarm which alerts the caregiver when the person with Alzheimer's strays beyond a certain distance or past an alarmed door. These are the typical systems found in care facilities such as nursing homes or adult day centers.

The second is a tracking device which uses a small transmitter, typically pager size or larger, attached to the wrist, ankle, or clothing of the person with Alzheimer's. The transmitter emits a continuous radio signal—if the person wanders away, the caregiver sets out after him or her with a handheld portable receiver about the size of an old-fashioned walkie-talkie. When the receiver is pointed in the direction of the lost person, it emits a beep which grows louder the closer the caregiver (or other person carrying the receiver) gets to the missing person wearing the transmitter. These transmitters are usually waterproof and can be worn 24 hours a day. Some can be set to emit their signal when the wearer leaves a certain perimeter, or safety range. Their range usually extends a few hundred yards to a mile or so. For an additional cost, some companies selling these products link the transmitter to a 24-hour central station—if the person wearing the transmitter wanders beyond the prescribed perimeter and the caregiver does not reset the receiver (as you would a home or office alarm system), a "central monitoring station" can page the caregiver or other family member (who must be wearing the required pager), call consenting neighbors, or the local police.

The third, and more potentially useful to help resolve wandering cases in the community, is a more sophisticated tracking device which uses the satellite-based Global Positioning System (GPS) in combination with the cellular technology used in mobile phones. With these GPS-based personal locator systems, the patient wears a tracking device somewhat larger than a pager which can be activated if the patient is reported missing. In its potential use to track Alzheimer patients, the device emits a signal that bounces off orbiting communications satellites to a "central monitoring station," which can notify caregivers that the patient is missing. The central monitoring station can also relay to police the real-time latitude and longitude coordinates determined by the satellite.

There are problems with these types of GPS-based locator systems. They currently require a great deal of energy to transmit and receive their signals (although their battery life continues to improve). They have for years been available in automobiles, where battery, transmitter, and receiver size is not such an issue. Their use with people requires miniaturization, which remains an issue—the smaller the battery, the shorter the transmission life of the device. Secondly, GPS requires simultaneous coordination of the view from 3 satellites, and performs with greater accuracy when the target of the GPS signal is in an open area with the transmitter (or "tag") in view. This becomes problematic in the concrete canyons of the typical city, just as it does in areas of dense foliage—where, as the Koester research and our own case studies indicate, the Alzheimer's wanderer is often found. And finally, to date the GPS-based locator technology is also not yet cost effective for general use among people with Alzheimer's disease. As the research (described below) will show, caregiver focus groups have indicated a willingness to purchase such a locator device if its costs are kept to about a $100 one-time startup charge and about $20 a month thereafter (Mellilo & Futrell, 1998). Systems dependent on GPS are currently more expensive.

However, a new wrinkle in the evolution of personal locator technology developed with a mandate issued by the Federal Communications Commission (FCC), calling for all cell phone providers to offer the currently operable Enhanced 911 (E911) phone system for home phones to all cell phone customers. (The FCC's initial, perhaps ambitious, target date of October 31, 2001 has been extended to 2005.) But this mandate has given rise to competition in the high-tech electrical engineering world to develop a miniaturized, cheap, accurate, energy efficient, and nonlabor intensive cellular-based personal locator device not necessarily dependent on GPS. Some companies are attempting to make the leap, based on the FCC mandate, to adapt the E911 system currently being developed for cell phones for cellular-based tracking purposes as well. Various federal agencies have invested funds in this high-tech effort (including the Departments of Energy, Defense, and Justice, and the National Institutes of Health and the National Institute on Aging—this last specifically for tracking people with memory impairments). One company began demonstrations of its system late in 1999, using its own self-standing cell towers. (This technology is referenced below in Melillo & Futrell, 1998.) Full deployment nationwide would involve use of a certain number of existing cell towers across the country, or globe. More appears later in the chapter on how this system, when deployed, would operate in the case of an Alzheimer's wanderer. First, a general review of the literature on personal locator technology.

Several research studies have examined the feasibility of caregivers using wandering alert devices, and found positive results. Melillo and Futrell (1998) surveyed 250 Alzheimer's caregivers by mail about wandering experiences and the possible use of a Patient Locator Unit (PLU), "a device consisting of a small, low-cost electronic bracelet [used] to quickly locate patients within a range of 6 to 10 miles using a single 25 kHz frequency allocation. The core properties of this technology are high accuracy, long battery life, and low-cost base station and mobile units." The researchers found that nearly all of the caregivers indicated that there was a need for a PLU and most were willing to pay for it. More specifically, the majority of caregivers were willing to pay a $100 initial fee and $10 to $20 a month for such a device. Caregivers felt that the PLU would give them a "greater peace of mind . . . help increase the control of the caregiver, and make it easier to locate wandering patients."

Similarly, in a feasibility study of 24 patients, McShane and colleagues (1998) found that 9 participants consistently used a tracking device as part of the research study. With 2 patients, it was successfully used in a search. One patient was injured by a passing vehicle when he got lost out of range of the device. Seven percent of the caregivers surveyed (N = 99) thought they could have benefitted from using the device at the time of the survey, and a further 11% could have benefitted at an earlier point in their illness.

Altus and colleagues (2000) evaluated the Mobile Locater, an electronic device using radio frequency designed to help caregivers quickly locate a missing patient. The 6-month study followed 7 users of the device and included an opinion survey of family caregivers, professional caregivers, and search and rescue workers. Survey results showed that respondents were positively impressed by the device, but identified cost as a potential drawback. Cost was more a barrier to use among family caregivers, who were less likely to use the device than were search and rescue personnel, which should serve as a note of caution about placing the burden of finding missing patients on families rather than on law enforcement and other properly equipped agencies.

An advantage of using wanderer control technology, however, is that such systems do not restrict freedom of movement. Zagami and colleagues (1998) remind us that "the goal of location management for wandering is not to totally confine the patients, because it is considered desirable to give patients both a sense of independence and the opportunity to exercise. Rather, the goal is to ensure the safety of the wandering individual, and to lessen the caregiver burden."

While many argue that cost is a barrier, others suggest that an advantage to using technology-based interventions is that they may be more humane and cost effective than institutional care. The cost of such systems may also be more manageable when compared with "the human cost and the expense of the search teams" (Coombs, 1994, p. 207).

While technological interventions might be less familiar than other prevention possibilities, they do address caregiver concerns for both safety and personal autonomy. They can sometimes reduce risk by finding the missing patient more quickly, allow the patient a greater degree of freedom, and help lessen caregiver anxiety.

And while there are merits to using such systems, especially as they continue to evolve and improve, there are also problems with wandering locator devices. The greatest drawback to the effectiveness of any device is misuse, including disengaging or ignoring alarms. The problem of false alarms or alarms that are not sufficiently responsive can lead to such misuse. It is very important that devices be reliable.

With all current locator systems, the person with Alzheimer's wears a device or an electronic "tag" which can be detected. As indicated earlier, many people with Alzheimer's disease or a related disorder may not tolerate wearing these devices, and may be quite persistent in attempting to remove bracelets or tags (McShane, Hope, & Wilkinson, 1994; Silverstein & Salmons, 1996).

A further problem with using this technology is that caregivers have to be able to respond to the alert and possibly search for the missing person. For caregivers who are not readily mobile, these technological strategies may not prove effective. For someone with Alzheimer's who lives alone, McShane and colleagues (1998) point out the greatly increased risk of injury or death because of the length of time before their absence is noted. The authors suggest that "regular home visits, together with a transmitting device which remained attached semipermanently, on a wristwatch strap for example, coupled with a locating system which did not require active searching would be required. A system of sensors within the home could alert a distant carer to a change in the pattern of someone's activities which might be useful to provide early warning of the patient's absence."

As was noted in McShane and colleagues (1998) feasibility study, in order to have a locator system in place caregivers have to recognize the risk of getting lost before it happens. If caregivers believe the risk of getting lost is small or that the person with Alzheimer's will only walk in the immediate vicinity, such a precaution is not likely to be regarded as important.

Financial burden or perceived burden is often cited as a deterrent to use of locator technology, but research suggests that the cost of these devices is often less expensive than the cost of searching or, due to the increased potential for serious injury, the cost of medical treatment or hospitalization (Coombs, 1994).

Technical issues may also serve as barriers to using personal locator systems. Any system or alarm requires training, and the more sophisticated locator systems require computer mapping software. For caregivers, this may prove to be problematic. Coombs points out that "computer use is not a way of life for many seniors. . . . In many cases, the best rehabilitative approach is the minimalist approach, wherein the devices that are easiest to use and the fewest devices are offered. Clinical experience has shown that introducing one aid at a time, and allowing the person to gain some skill at using it, promotes easier acceptance of a second aid" (p. 207). Although we realize that barriers to computer use among older people are not what they were thought to be several years ago, for elderly caregivers who may have arthritis or poor eyesight, the screens and buttons associated with locator devices and technology may be problematic.

And while some suggest that this technology might help the person with Alzheimer's live at home for as long as possible, others suggest that the work connected with using it is a burden for caregivers. McShane and colleagues (1998) offers the following comments:

> Looking after people with dementia is labor intensive. It is tempting to think that this form of electronic device would enable people to be kept at home who would otherwise require institutional care. Our experience suggests otherwise. Not only does someone have to ensure that the patient is wearing the device, but the recognition that someone has left their home or has not returned when expected also requires someone "on the ground." Furthermore, someone needs to do the searching. . . . There are barriers to the use of tracking devices which no amount of technological innovation will resolve. Someone needs to recognize that the patient is at risk, and both informal and professional carers may need educating about this. Someone will always need to ensure that the device is attached to the patient and go and fetch them. The use of electronic tracking devices is warranted for carefully selected patients with dementia. Technological developments may yet allow more patients to benefit. However, continuing research will help to temper excessive enthusiasm for a technical solution to a social problem (pp. 561–563).

Additionally, the user friendliness of a personal locator system goes a long way toward ensuring that the system will actually be used. Before going high tech, it is wise for caregivers to ask some basic but critical questions:

- Does the system work well in all weather conditions?
- Has it actually prevented or reduced patient wandering? What are some of the seller's success stories? Failures?

- Does it break down? How often?
- How are repairs accomplished? How are replacement parts obtained?
- How frequent is service required?
- How difficult is installation?
- What is the cost of maintaining the system? Cost of batteries, electricity, triggers?

Further, the logistical difficulties associated with search and rescue efforts cannot be overstated. It is unrealistic to expect an 80-year-old woman to hunt through the woods for her missing husband with Alzheimer's disease while waving a bulky receiver, as might be the case with some existing locator technology. It may be just as unrealistic to expect the hundreds of local police departments in each state, which generally control searches in their jurisdiction, to purchase these receivers in the expectation that: 1) caregivers will then purchase the transmitters (or a third party donate them to caregivers in large numbers); and 2) they will have trained personnel to maintain the receivers and that these personnel will also be available to deploy the receivers in a uniform and timely manner. It is also likely that any state police department or county sheriff's office would want to enhance its budget before committing to handling a labor intensive and time-consuming electronic personal locator system on behalf of local police departments.

On the other hand, as referenced earlier, there is competition in the high-tech electrical engineering world to develop a miniaturized, cheap, accurate, energy efficient, and nonlabor-intensive cellular-based personal locator system not necessarily dependent on GPS. Such a system would work in much the same way GPS-dependent locator devices work, but would probably be smaller, more accurate, longer-lived, and more affordable. In a practical application of this emerging technology, the Alzheimer's patient would wear a watch-size transmitter on the arm, ankle, or elsewhere. A responsible source—a police officer, a family or professional caregiver—on discovering that the patient is missing, would call a central monitoring station (the transmitter might also be set to activate when the patient leaves a given perimeter, or is gone for a certain length of time). The central monitoring station, operating from an Internet site, inputs specific codes—similar to dialing a pager or cell phone number—triggering a signal to the patient's miniaturized transmitter via cell tower equipment in the area where the patient is reported missing; the patient's transmitter responds, emitting a signal detected by the cell tower, which relays latitude and longitude coordinates back to the central monitoring station, where they are plotted with simple desktop mapping software; the central monitoring station then notifies the police or caregiver of the lost patient's specific location, which could, in theory, be tracked continuously.

Emerging technology has the real potential to save lives. As mentioned earlier in the chapter, there is financial support available through various state and federal programs for memory-impaired elders who could benefit from it. And some personal locator systems may meet the criteria caregivers have indicated they want in such technology: affordability, practicality, and accuracy (Mellilo & Futrell, 1998). Until such a system is fully engineered and marketed, however, our best advice to caregivers who might purchase an expensive alarm system or tracking device is to first spend their money on care in an adult day center or on other types of respite. As much of the literature on tracking and location devices for people with dementia indicates, no technological solution will fully resolve social problems like wandering behavior. Even when the best personal locator technology does arrive, meets caregivers' criteria (and possibly complements programs like Safe Return), the bottom line for people with dementia is still going to involve therapeutic care and supervision.

In Their Own Words: Caregivers Talk About Police Involvement

And they knew that there was no little son at her age, so they called the police and they came and . . . I guess through the name they knew where to bring her. One of the policemen that brought her here just went into her house and sat and talked with her so when our neighbor came, they were talking. For weeks after, she would still tell people about it and how the police had to bring her home, so she wasn't happy about it.

The first time I was at work and I got a phone call (from police). Our neighbor up the street is a police lieutenant, and two of my kids worked at the police station when they were going to school so they know the name and the family and everything.

He would disappear . . . I would go looking and eventually would call the police and the police would come and find him. Once he was in some bushes. The police had spent all night looking for him but they didn't find him.

In the last 2 years, it might have been anywhere between 15 and 20 times. The police were involved at least two-thirds of those times.

He went to the bank, drew out money, didn't have the bank book but they knew him at the bank—when you first started talking to him you would think he was okay. He told them that he had won money in the lottery and that he needed the money to go to New York to collect his winnings and he would share his winnings with the bank teller if she would give him $100. He convinced this lady that she should give him this $100 and he went off to New York! He went to New York! We still don't know how he got there! But the police brought him back. He was gone maybe a weekend, or it was a couple of days. And the police finally brought him back. We had called the police and my mother was just frantic! Because we had no idea where he went and we still don't know the whole story. To think that he had gone that far!

One time, he took off and he must have walked about 10 miles! He would disappear . . . I would go looking and eventually would call the police and the police would come and find him. Once, the police had spent all night looking for him but they didn't find him.

It was only he and I down there (in Florida) and he was gone for hours! And a fellow who used to be my boss saw him and called me and said, "I just saw your husband," and it was like 3 or 4 miles from where we were. And I was really panicky with no support system down there so he said he'd get in the car and go back and I'd get in the car and head this way. We found him. I saw the police car first. It was dark by then. And what had happened, he tripped on the curb and broke his nose. And so I take him to the hospital in Florida and he was just plain exhausted, disoriented. So that was probably the scariest because I was in Florida and I didn't know my way around down there.

He went out and didn't have any shoes on. I don't know where he went but when we found him his feet were bleeding. He had to go to the hospital. The police found him that time and brought him back. He had been wandering for quite some time before they caught up with him.

Chapter 6

Long-Term Care Providers

We want to believe that if we entrust our family member in a formalized care setting such as in adult day health care, assisted living, or a nursing facility, that that care provider will assure that the individual with dementia will be safe. Unfortunately, many facilities cannot provide that assurance and if they do make that claim, we would encourage you to ask for evidence:

- How many elopements have there been in the past year?
- What were the consequences of those elopements? How quickly were people found, by whom, and in what shape?
- What protocols exist for responding to incidences of elopement?
- How often do individuals with dementia *attempt* to elope but are stopped in time?
- What specialized training have staff members received in dementia care? What level(s) of staff members have received training?
- What activities are especially directed toward individuals who display a tendency to wander?
- Have any environmental modifications been made to therapeutically support individuals with dementia?
- Is the facility aware of the Safe Return program that is sponsored by the national Alzheimer's Association in cooperation with the U.S. Justice Department? Are clients in adult day care or residents in assisted living or nursing facilities registered in Safe Return?

Facilities that "get it" should be able to respond to your inquiries with well thought out plans. Facilities that say, "Wandering has never been a problem here" are likely to be in denial or, perhaps, are heavy users of physical or chemical restraints.

Wandering episodes that become more frequent and catastrophic are one of the reasons that the caregiver of the community-residing individual with dementia makes the decision to institutionalize. The caregiver makes this decision of last resort with the assumption that an institutional environment will be safer for the individual with dementia. Safety, however, cannot be assumed.

Researchers have documented for at least 20 years or more that wandering and becoming lost from an institutional residence is a regular occurrence. Kennedy (1993) noted that best estimates indicate that, "each week, at least one resident of this nation's nursing home care facilities will wander away from the premises to meet death by exposure, starvation, drowning, falling, or motor vehicle accident" (p. 170). Dickinson, McLain-Kark, and Marshall-Baker (1995) observed that "unsafe exiting in dementia care units due to wandering presents problems for residents . . . " (p. 127). They noted Burnside's 1981 finding that "approximately 20% of staff employed at long-term care facilities reported at least one incident where wandering resulted in injury or death" (ibid).

Beyond the screening questions that are offered on the previous page, how can you measure how well a facility is likely to manage wandering behavior? Two factors that are critical to consider are the physical environment and the level of staff training. Considering the relationship between environment and staff training, the goal of the long-term care industry should be to place well-trained staff in a therapeutically dementia-friendly environment. Cohen-Mansfield, Werner, Marx, and Freedman (1991) note that "nursing home residents who pace or wander present significant management problems for caregivers" (p. M77), and they encourage staff to consider pacing a reflection of good physical health and a behavior that should not be restricted but rather encouraged under optimal environmental conditions. This positive orientation to a high-risk behavior is not likely to come naturally to staff and suggests a need for specialized training. The negative orientation is likely to be a dependence on physical and chemical restraints. Although the latter is becoming less the norm with an increasing number of nursing homes becoming "restraint-free" and utilizing alternatives to restraints (Miles, 1996).

The optimal situation should be to have staff who are specially trained and working in a therapeutically supportive environment. Where the optimal situation does not exist, then the short-term goals of facilities should be to have well-trained staff compensate for a less than optimally therapeutic environment and vice versa, that is, a strong environment that compensates for staff that have minimal training. This relationship is portrayed in Figure 6.1 below. A staff that is aware of the specialized needs of the residents on their unit and provides appropriate activities and close supervision to residents with dementia, including daily walks outdoors, may be able to minimize the effect of an environment that has poor exit control. Similarly, a staff that is not in tune with the specialized needs of residents with dementia and does not provide close supervision may avoid potentially catastrophic situations by working in an environment that has strong exit control. In addition, Kennedy (1993) reported on staffing ratios for working with residents with dementia and suggested that 1:5 would be ideal; 1:6 or 7 would be adequate; and 1:8 or more patients would be insufficient (p. 174). However, increased staffing alone does not sufficiently compensate for the need for specialized training and environmental modifications.

ENVIRONMENT

	NOT SUPPORTIVE	**HIGHLY SUPPORTIVE**
MINIMALLY TRAINED STAFF	*Poor*	*Good*
WELL-TRAINED STAFF	*Good*	*Best*

FIGURE 6.1 Level of staff training and supportive environment.

The level of staffing and specialized training received is something that you can observe and inquire about. The environment, however, requires a trained eye to know what and when to observe. What exactly makes an environment therapeutic and supportive? Zeisel, et al., defined eight environmental factors that might therapeutically influence behavior of individuals with Alzheimer's disease in an institutional setting. Those eight factors are: exit control, wandering paths, individual away spaces, common space structure, outdoor freedom, residential scale, autonomy support, and sensory comprehension. With Zeisel's Environment-Behavior (E-B) checklist, it becomes possible to walk through a facility and objectively assess it for the degree its environment therapeutically responds to behaviors associated with dementia. Wandering is the behavior that we are focusing on here, but Zeisel, et al., also looked at depression, sleep disorders, social withdrawal, delusions and hallucinations, misidentification syndrome, aggression, anxiety, and agitation. Readers who are interested in a nonpharmacological approach for managing behaviors of individuals with dementia are encouraged to read Zeisel, J., Hyde, J., & Levkoff, S. (March/April 1994), Best practices: An environment-behavior model (E-B) for Alzheimer's special care units in *The American Journal of Alzheimer's Care and Related Disorders & Research*, pp. 4–21, and Chapter 8 of this book. We will focus on three of the environmental influences that specifically relate to managing wandering behavior: exit control, wandering paths, and outdoor space.

The Environmental Dimensions That Impact Wandering

Exit control relates to the boundary conditions of each facility: the surrounding walls, fences, and doors, and how they are locked or otherwise control how people come and go. Wandering paths are defined as the circulation space the residents use for moving around. Outdoor freedom is the residents' access to common areas out of doors and the way these places support residents' needs. It is important to note that regulations vary from state to state and may impact the ability of a facility to respond to the implementation of design criteria that would be dementia friendly.

The full E-B checklist is presented and described in Hearthstone Alzheimer Care (1998), supported by a grant from the National Institute on Aging (AG12343), Hearthstone: Lexington, MA. Elements of the E-B checklist are presented below:

Exit control

The observer is looking for the level of obtrusiveness or the degree to which the location of doors influences the chance that residents will notice them. A facility that has a high level of exit control will have signals and other control devices—such as keypads—that keep the exits well controlled with few delays in warning signals. Doors, door handles, and security devices will be minimally visible, or unobtrusive, thus not providing residents with visual invitations to leave the unit or facility. This means that the residents in such units are safe as well as minimally attracted to the visual invitation to leave presented by a door. The exits are secured with little or no delay. The exits are designed so that residents are unaware of the doors themselves, locks, or security devices. A facility with a low level of exit control would have residents exiting on their own or shadowing visitors as they exit the unit. There are few barriers to exiting. Responsibility is on the staff to retrieve residents who elope. State fire regulations may dictate the type of signage, locking device, and windows required on exit doors.

Location of the exit door: The location influences the inevitability of running into and/or noticing door(s). The exit door that is at the end of a straight hallway is likely to beckon the individual forward. It is a clear destination. In contrast, an exit door that is in a common room off of a main hallway, so the individual finds an activity or destination as he or she exits off the hallway to a common room, may be less drawn to the exit from the common room. Ideally, the exit off the common room is to a therapeutic garden and outdoor wandering path. The main point is not to have the exit door "cue" the individual toward it.

- ❐ Exit door is at the end of a straight hallway.
- ❐ Exit door is at the end of a short alcove.
- ❐ Exit door is on the sidewall of hallway.
- ❐ Exit door is in the common room.

Foot traffic: Exit doors on busy, well-traveled hallways pose a greater threat to the individual with dementia than exit doors on less frequently traveled hallways. Staff and visitors going on and off the unit are constantly drawing attention to the door and may be inadvertently "inviting" residents to follow them.

- ❐ Exit door is on a frequently traveled path.
- ❐ Exit door is on a moderately traveled path.
- ❐ Exit door is on an infrequently traveled path.

Attraction of the exit door: Intuitively, exit doors should look different than nonexit doors. But with dementia, the goal is to have them look similar to nonexit doors and preferably, to look like the wall. You do not want the exit door to attract attention like a magnet. The observer is looking for the degree to which doors leading out of the unit resemble other nonexit doors.

- ❐ Exit door leading out of the unit is completely different from nonexit door and "stands out."

- ❒ Exit door is very different from nonexit door but "does not stand out."
- ❒ Exit door is somewhat different from nonexit door.
- ❒ Exit door is precisely the same as nonexit door.
- ❒ Exit door is camouflaged.

Signage on exit door: Too many signs on the door may encourage the individual to approach the door. The door becomes a center of attention because the signs make it interesting. The observer is looking at the degree to which objects attached to the exit door attracts residents' attention to that door.

- ❒ There are more than two signs on the exit door:
- ❒ There are one or two signs on the exit door.
- ❒ There are no signs on the exit door.

Hardware on exit door: Door handles, knobs, and bars made of shiny metal or elaborate designs may become objects of interest and attract residents toward them. Simplicity is safer.

- ❒ There is much visible hardware on the exit door.
- ❒ There is some visible hardware on the exit door.
- ❒ There is no visible hardware on the exit door.

Panic bar: The panic bar is meant to attract, and regulations may dictate that it must appear a particular way. Yet, the more its appearance stands out, the more dangerous it becomes for the individual with dementia. It serves as one more element that "draws" them to an exit door.

- ❒ There is a full panic fire hardware bar on the exit door.
- ❒ There is a nonpanic fire hardware bar on the exit door.
- ❒ There is no panic or fire hardware bar on the exit door.

Opacity: The concern here is that the resident will be drawn to whatever is on the other side of the door. That area may not be safe. Thus, the observer is looking for the degree to which the ability to see through to the other side of the door (opaqueness) attracts residents to the exit door.

- ❒ The exit door is all glass.
- ❒ The exit door has large windows.
- ❒ There is a small window in the exit door.

- ❒ There are slats in the exit door for airflow.
- ❒ The exit door is a solid door.

Use of space on other side of exit door: If the resident does exit, how safe is the area on the other side? The observer is looking at the degree to which the character and use of the space on the other side of the exit door tempts the residents to elope.

- ❒ The space on the other side of the exit door is highly active and full of people.
- ❒ The space on the other side of the exit door is often used, but not always.
- ❒ The space on the other side of the exit door is in use about half the time.
- ❒ The space on the other side of the exit door is only occasionally used.
- ❒ The space on the other side of the exit door is never used.

Safety risk outside of exit door: What is the level of concern for serious consequences in case an individual with dementia does elope? The observer is looking for the degree to which elopement through the exit door presents a safety risk to the residents.

- ❒ Exit door opens to an extremely unsafe area such as a busy street.
- ❒ Exit door opens to a moderately unsafe area such as an enclosed garden with a fence that may be climbed.
- ❒ Exit door opens to a somewhat safe area such as into another part of the facility where staff may or may not know residents from another unit.
- ❒ Exit door opens to a moderately safe area such as into another unit where staff is familiar with the residents outside of their unit.
- ❒ Exit door opens to a safe area such as an enclosed garden that has been planned for safety and is supervised.

Locking devices and alarms: What type of locking device or alarm is on the exit door? The observer is looking for the degree to which the door-locking device physically prevents elopement.

- ❒ There is no lock or alarm on the exit door (a "no exit" sign does not count as a lock).
- ❒ An alarm sounds when the exit door is opened but there is no locking device.
- ❒ There is an intermittent self-locking system where resident wears a band that triggers locking mechanism when exit door is approached.

- ❐ The exit door has a delayed signal alarm device such as a keypad.
- ❐ The exit door is alarmed and kept locked.

Signal delays: Is a signal delay in use on the exit door? Does too much time pass before an alarm is sounded?

- ❐ There is no buzzer or alarm on the exit door.
- ❐ The alarm rings after 15 seconds or more of pushing the exit door.
- ❐ The alarm signal is activated after 3 to 15 seconds of pushing the exit door.
- ❐ The alarm signal is activated in 3 seconds or less of pushing the exit door.
- ❐ The alarm signal is activated every time the exit door is opened or touched.

Signal sounds: Loud sounds can upset the individual with dementia and cause agitation. The goal is to have signals that are meaningful to the staff but do not cause disruption for the individual. The observer is looking for the degree to which the type of alarm signal attracts the residents' attention.

- ❐ The alarm signal on the exit door makes a loud noise or a visual signal.
- ❐ The alarm signal on the exit door makes a moderate noise or visual signal.
- ❐ The alarm signal on the exit door makes a soft noise or visual signal.
- ❐ The alarm signal on the exit door makes a soft "click" as the resident approaches.
- ❐ The alarm signal on the exit door has no sign, noise, or visual signal apparent to residents.

Time missing from unit: When elopements do occur, how are they handled? How much time passes before the individual is found? Specifically, ask staff about last elopement or attempted elopement. How much time had elapsed between the time the resident eloped or attempted to elope and was retrieved? You do not want to hear that there was an indefinite time before the resident was safely back on the unit (or that the resident is not back at all).

- ❐ The resident is brought back by the police or nonstaff person.
- ❐ The resident is brought back by a staff member.
- ❐ The resident is slowly dissuaded by an alarmed door.
- ❐ The resident is quickly dissuaded by a delayed door.

- ❐ The resident attempts but is unable to elope because of a locked door.
- ❐ Staff intervention is not needed to prevent resident elopement from exit door.

Wandering paths

The observer is looking for the degree to which the shape of the wandering path reduces the number of decision points. A facility with a high value on wandering paths is one in which corridors and other pathways in the unit and in any enclosed resident outdoor space are: easy to use, represent a continuous trip, and provide residents using corridors and pathways with understandable visual cues and interesting events that support therapeutic walking. Cues are indicators of appropriate behavior. A sign is an overt cue indicating where to go (bathroom) or how to behave (no smoking). A less overt cue might be a change in floor covering helping residents sense the difference between a hallway and a bedroom.

The more elements of interest along a pathway (views, artwork, objects), the more interesting the trip is for residents. This in turn provides residents with a motivation to stop and attend to an object or view outside the window, and eventually move to another destination along the pathway. Low value for wandering paths within a unit would be a facility with a limited and uninteresting corridor as the only place that residents might use to walk. There are likely to be regulatory issues that vary from state to state regarding the construction of wandering paths.

Observe the layout of the unit. Is it a straight corridor? Does it have alcoves on either side that alter the straight path? Does it have small alcoves in the corners or is it "T-shaped?" Is it basically a square or rectangle? Does it seem like a centipede with lots of directions to branch off? Is part of it inside the unit and part outside? Or is it a continuous path or circular loop?

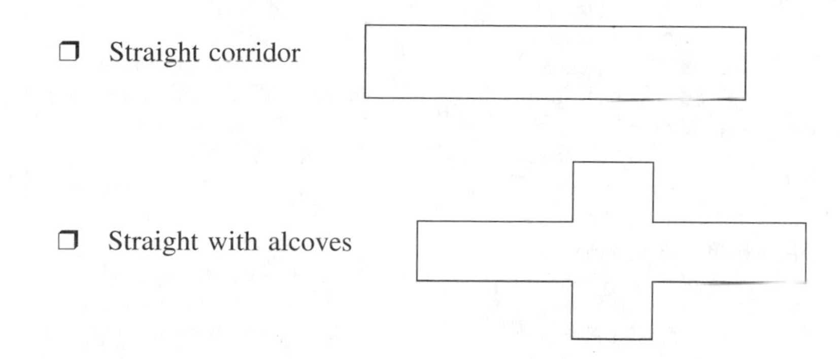

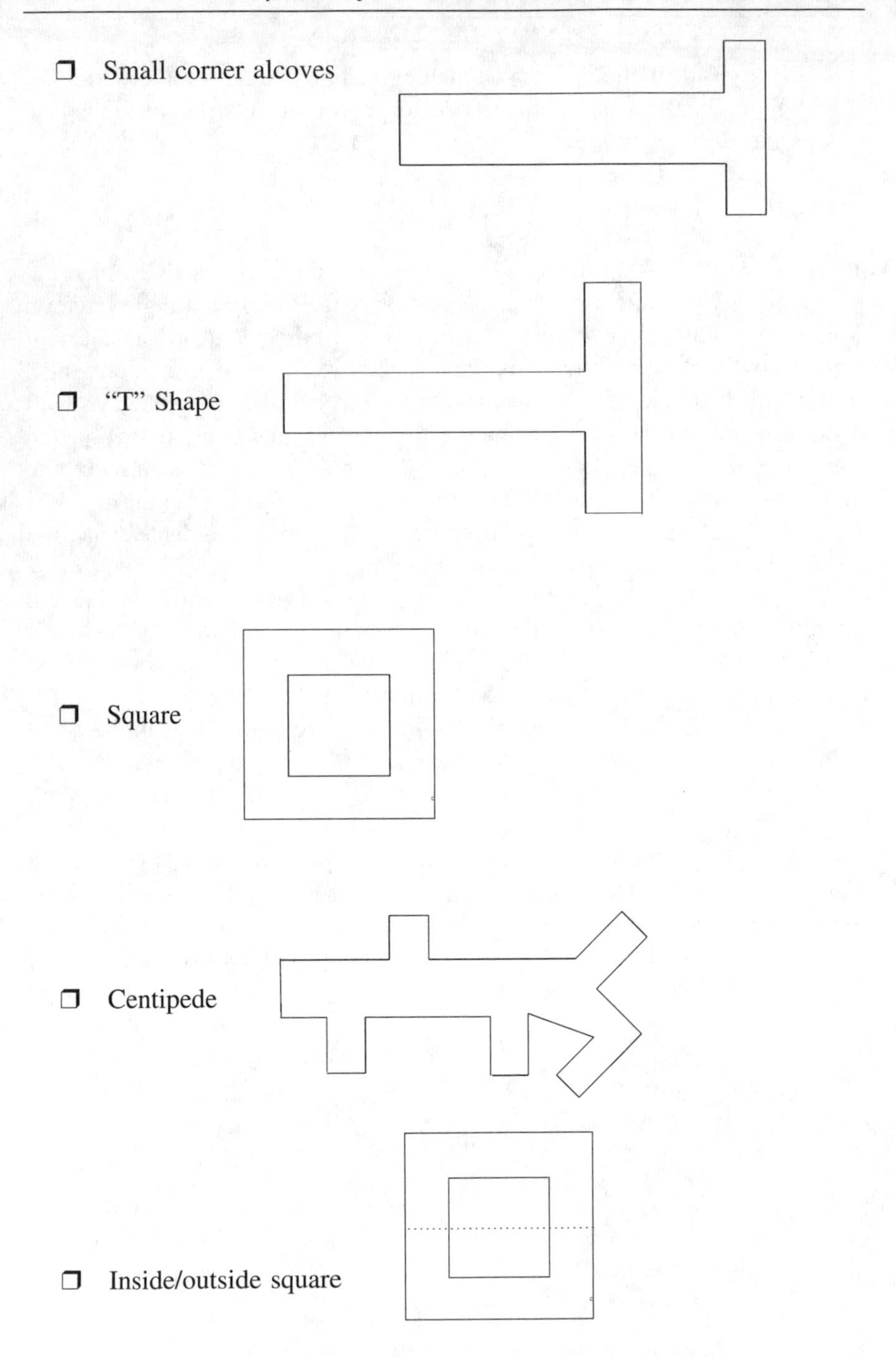
❒ Small corner alcoves
❒ "T" Shape
❒ Square
❒ Centipede
❒ Inside/outside square

❐ Circle/oval

Turning potential: The unit becomes the individual's home and neighborhood combined. Is there someplace to walk? And when he or she reaches a destination, is there a clear path to the second destination? Destinations can be spaces or elements such as benches, plants, pictures, activity spaces, dining rooms, and nursing stations. The degree to which pathway social space and element locations increase turning potential at ends of corners of walking paths is important.

- ❐ Turning potential is low (dead-ends at end of corridor/corner with few views).
- ❐ Turning potential is medium to low (few turning elements such as wall art or views).
- ❐ Turning potential is medium (some dead-ends, some active areas).
- ❐ Turning potential is medium to high (many turning elements such as wall art, and views to side of corridor).
- ❐ Turning potential is high (activity spaces at corridor ends and corners).

Degree to which environment provides orienting landmarks: Where do the paths lead? Are there defining landmarks? Does the destination have a purpose?

- ❐ Pathways lead nowhere (i.e., blank wall, locked door) no matter where resident is headed.
- ❐ Some of the pathway directions provide destination purposes.
- ❐ Half of the pathway directions provide destination purposes.
- ❐ Most of the pathway directions provide destination purposes.
- ❐ Every place along the pathway provides a destination with purpose.

Degree to which pathway provides confusion or clarity: Clear pathways are important to minimize falls and avoid increased confusion. Clutter can also be excess furniture and equipment. Many units have limited storage areas, so finding medical trays, wheelchairs, and maintenance equipment stored in the hallway may not be unusual. Still, it presents a problem for the individual with dementia.

- ❒ Pathway is very cluttered.
- ❒ Pathway is somewhat cluttered.
- ❒ Pathway is neither cluttered nor orderly.
- ❒ Pathway is somewhat orderly.
- ❒ Pathway is very orderly.

Number of "window-shopping" elements along the path:

- ❒ There are no views, wall art, or objects to see along the path.
- ❒ There are very few views, wall art, or objects to see along the path.
- ❒ There are occasional views, wall art, or objects to see along the path.
- ❒ There are many views, wall art, or objects to see along the path.
- ❒ Views, wall art, or objects to see are continuous along the path.

Outdoor space

Look for the degree to which a facility's outdoor space is immediately accessible to residents, and the extent to which this outdoor space is especially planned for use by dementia residents. A facility with a high ranking on outdoor space has an immediately adjacent secure outdoor space on the same level as the dementia unit, where caregivers perceive the space to be safe and secure enough that residents are given largely independent access to the space. In addition, the outdoor space has physical elements that are designed to support Alzheimer's residents to function effectively outdoors. Such elements include planters that enable residents to have contact with soil, nonpoisonous plants, and visibility of the unit so that residents can easily find their way back. In particular, having the outdoor space on the same level and with staff offices located to allow easy surveillance will maximize the residents' use of such space at their own discretion. A facility that provides residents only limited and occasional access to an outdoor area that has not been designed for use by individuals with dementia, ranks lowest on outdoor space. Residents placed on higher floors have limited access to outdoor space. Financial output is necessary to design a therapeutic garden space and to erect fencing.

Degree of enclosure:

- ❒ The outdoor space is not enclosed. It is a public space like a sidewalk.
- ❒ There is only a symbolic, not effective, enclosure like low hedges, to the outdoor space.
- ❒ There is a low fence or some plantings, but the outdoor space is not locked.

- ❒ The outdoor space is locked but residents could elope over fence or through hedges.
- ❒ The outdoor space has high enclosures and is locked.

Consequences of elopement:

- ❒ The area beyond the outdoor space is extremely unsafe, like a busy street.
- ❒ The area beyond the outdoor space is moderately unsafe, such as an enclosed garden with a fence that might be climbed.
- ❒ The area beyond the outdoor space presents a low risk of negative consequences for the resident but is not really safe, such as another area that is on the grounds of the facility.
- ❒ The area beyond the outdoor space is moderately safe, such as an area that is on the grounds of the facility and is supervised.
- ❒ The area beyond the outdoor space is completely enclosed and is supervised.

Dedicated space for individuals with dementia only:

- ❒ The outdoor space is shared with nondementia residents.
- ❒ The outdoor space is not dedicated but is used primarily with residents with dementia.
- ❒ The outdoor space is dedicated for use with residents with dementia.

Degree of direct accessibility from the unit:

- ❒ The outdoor space is far from the unit.
- ❒ The outdoor space is accessible from the unit only by an elevator.
- ❒ The outdoor space is near the unit, but does not have direct access from the unit.
- ❒ The outdoor space is directly accessible from the unit.

Frequency of use:

- ❒ The outdoor space is never used.
- ❒ The outdoor space is rarely used (about once a week).
- ❒ The outdoor space is sometimes used (2–3 times a week).
- ❒ The outdoor space is frequently used (4–6 times a week).
- ❒ The outdoor space is used daily.

Door to outside space:

- ❒ The door to the outside space is generally kept locked.
- ❒ The door to the outside space is unlocked only on occasion, i.e., during a scheduled activity time.
- ❒ The door to the outside space is sometimes unlocked, usually for a half day either a.m. or p.m.
- ❒ The door to the outside space is unlocked daily for a specified time period such as 8 a.m. to 8 p.m.
- ❒ The door to the outside space is unlocked 24 hours a day.

Opacity of the door to the outdoor space:

- ❒ The door to the outside space is solid without windows.
- ❒ The door to the outside space may be seen through if the resident strains.
- ❒ The door to the outside space has small windows.
- ❒ The door to the outside space is screened or has slightly obscured windows.
- ❒ The door to the outside space is easily seen through with large windows or all glass.

Policy or practice related to the outdoor space:

- ❒ The resident must always be escorted to the outdoor space.
- ❒ The resident is sometimes escorted to the outdoor space.
- ❒ The resident is never escorted to the outdoor space.

Level of supervision in use of outdoor space:

- ❒ The resident is never supervised in the outdoor space.
- ❒ The resident is sometimes supervised in the outdoor space.
- ❒ The resident is always supervised in the outdoor space.

Degree to which the design of the open space supports the needs, frailties, and abilities of residents with Alzheimer's disease or a related disorder:

- ❒ Surfaces, other than pathways
- ❒ Pathway surface
- ❒ Clarity of pathway as the place to walk

- ❒ Shade
- ❒ Outdoor furniture
- ❒ Activity areas
- ❒ Plants and planters

Conducting such an "environmental audit" can help staff and family members understand the strengths and limitations of their environment. Some things can be changed, others may require modifications that are too costly. In these situations, staff should have a heightened awareness of environmental concerns that could impact dementia care. Chapters 8 and 9 provide recommendations to agencies and facilities for how to meet environmental challenges with respect to wandering behavior.

Part III

Creating a Safe Environment

Introduction

Part III offers concrete suggestions for creating safe environments to address the constant risk of unsafe wandering behavior in the home, community, and long-term care facility. This is not about advocating for a "prisonlike" environment—this is about maximizing independence within the constraints of the disease process. Individuals with dementia move in and out of settings in the course of daily living and come in contact with a wide range of formal and informal care providers. The majority of the care providers are well-meaning, but many may not have specialized knowledge of managing wandering behavior.

Recommendations that apply to all settings are:

- Increased understanding of the risks of wandering behavior and strategies for minimizing serious consequences.
- Increased awareness of the physical environment and settings that can be therapeutic and supportive versus those settings that may present great risk and are not supportive.
- Increased acknowledgment of the need for supervision.

The sequence of chapters in this section takes the reader through the continuum of care from the home environment, to the community providers, and finally, to the long-term care facility. It is not a linear path—cognitively impaired elders who reside at home may also attend adult day health programs. In addition, cognitively impaired elders, like elders in general, are also likely to experience hospitalization. Thus, Chapter 8 devotes substantive discussion to recommendations for acute care providers.

Chapter 10 discusses the role of the "first responders," the police and search and rescue professionals who are faced with the consequences of an elopement. We acknowledge that even with the best of care under the supervision of the most informed professional or family member, and surrounded by an optimally supportive environment, wandering will occur. Our goal throughout this book has been to provide tools to try to minimize those occurrences. When a wandering episode does occur, we want the assurances that police and search and rescue personnel understand wandering behavior and the patterns that cognitively impaired individuals are likely to follow. Such knowledge can greatly assist the search effort. In addition, chapter 10 assists first responders in understanding the role of family members, professional care providers, and the Alzheimer's Association Safe Return program in locating the missing elder.

CHAPTER 7

The Home: Recommendations for Family Caregivers

In the following pages, we make recommendations and suggest strategies to help family caregivers create a safe home environment. A safe environment can assist families in coping with the difficulties that wandering presents, reduce its frequency, and minimize its catastrophic consequences.

We focus on recommended techniques to help the family caregiver cope with the problem of wandering and improve the safety of the home environment for three important reasons:

1. The family is more likely than formal care providers to be the primary caregiver.
2. Wandering episodes and attempts to wander often result in serious consequences such as injury, hospitalization, or placement in a nursing home.
3. There are safeguards that can be taken to minimize wandering episodes that are relatively easy and low cost to implement.

Note that there are suggestions for safety precautions in facilities which follow in chapter 8 that may be applicable to the home setting as well. In addition, social workers and geriatric care managers are advised to use these recommendations in their work with elders and their caregivers in the community.

The Family Is the Main Caregiver and the First Line of Defense

The majority of care of frail elders, including those with Alzheimer's disease or a related dementia, is provided in the community and by the family (Horowitz, 1985; Kapp, 1995). In fact, "it (Alzheimer's disease) is often referred to as a family disease, because all members of the family are affected by it emotionally, financially, and socially" (Riekse & Holstege, 1996, p. 100). There are an estimated 2.4 to 3.1 million Alzheimer's disease caregivers in the United States (Schulz, O'Brien, Bookwala, & Fleissner, 1995). Moreover, a national survey conducted in 1993 indicates that approximately 19 million Americans say they have a family member with Alzheimer's or a related dementia, and 37 million know someone with the disease (Alzheimer's Association, 2002).

Throughout this book and again in this chapter, we convey what is known about wandering—that it is a common symptom of Alzheimer's disease, that anyone can experience the behavior, and that it often occurs without warning. Incidents of wandering, both episodes and attempts, can cause tremendous stress for the family. These occurrences may also result in serious or fatal injury.

Before turning to specific suggestions for creating a safe environment and coping with wandering in the home, there are several important points to keep in mind:

- Recognizing and acknowledging the struggles that family caregivers face is discussed in chapter 4. There are the difficulties associated with providing 24-hour supervision (which is often recommended as the most effective precaution for unsafe wandering behavior); the dilemma of wanting to preserve the family member's autonomy and independence while keeping them safe as well; the many competing demands and problems that family caregivers face on a daily basis; and the problems with safety techniques that are too difficult to implement, too expensive to afford, or too detrimental to the dignity of the family member with dementia. These struggles cannot be overlooked and many of the recommended strategies in the following pages have been informed by their realities.
- Despite the struggles mentioned above and detailed in chapter 4, it is also important to realize that all of those with dementia are at risk for unsafe wandering and that the consequences can be deadly. Despite the range of prevalence discussed earlier in chapter 2, many experts

agree that all people with dementia should be presumed to be at risk for wandering due to their cognitive deficits and unpredictable behavior (Coltharp, Richie, & Kaas, 1996; Flaherty & Raia, 1994). Any interventions or management strategies must also take this important perspective into account.

- Not every safety strategy will work for every person or family. In the following pages, we provide a menu of safety techniques for dealing with the problem of wandering. We encourage families to try different strategies and find the ones that work and are most effective for them. Caregivers often report having several interventions in place on an ongoing basis—this is a recommended way of dealing with the problem so that if one technique fails there are other safeguards in place. No one thing will work for everyone. We offer a range of possibilities. There is no single solution. Intervention must be multifaceted and individualized.

Recommended Management Strategies

Before we turn to specific recommended strategies for unsafe wandering, the overall idea is that prevention is the best solution. While there are various safety measures for when wandering has already occurred and the person with dementia is out or lost, most of the precautions in the following pages are aimed at preventing unsafe wandering from happening in the first place.

Handler (1988), and Pynoos and Ohta (1991) suggest that home adaptation is an important factor in managing the person with Alzheimer's disease in the community. However, family caregivers do not always comply with professional recommendations on home adaptation. Family caregivers need to be convinced of the effectiveness of a recommendation before they take steps to modify their home environment. Family caregivers also need to be in agreement with the professional that the target problem—in this case, wandering—is indeed serious enough to warrant modification (Silverstein & Hyde, 1997). In the same study, nurse practitioners made an average of 25 home adaptation recommendations to family caregivers based on an initial home assessment. Three of the top five recommendations dealt with concerns about potential wandering. The other two recommendations related to the potential for poisonous ingestion. The three recommendations related to wandering were: have copies of a current photo available, have individual with dementia wear an identification bracelet (specifically, a Safe Return bracelet), and install additional locks on exit doors.

Thus, our recommendations, like the professionals before us, are speaking as much to the "potential" for wandering as they do to the aftermath of a wandering episode. Wandering is, indeed, a serious behavior that warrants a serious response. It is with an eye toward the "potential for wandering" that our strategies should be considered.

We strongly recommend against employing a wait-and-see strategy that may result in having to respond to a crisis and we concur that "the best defense against wandering is to prevent it from happening" (Davis, 1991, p. 40). We also argue that the simplest precautions are often the best. The real key is to stop people before they reach the perimeter. There are inexpensive and easy ways of doing that which are highlighted in this chapter.

Strategies to protect individuals and families from the risks associated with wandering can be grouped as follows: 1) *environmental management strategies* that use assistive devices and techniques such as alarms, disguising doors, or putting locks very high or very low; 2) *community strategies* such as registering the person with Safe Return and notifying the local police; 3) *stimulation strategies* such as providing increased activity, chores, and other meaningful tasks during the day; and 4) *monitoring strategies* including walking with, following, or shadowing the person.

Environmental management strategies

Managing the environment includes considering both the outside surroundings as well as the interior of the home and should begin with a careful assessment of the two environments followed by the implementation of appropriate interventions.

The Outside Environment

- Review the environment in and around the home for possible hazards—swimming pools, dense foliage, tunnels, steep stairways, high balconies, and roadways where traffic tends to be heavy—and limit access to potentially dangerous areas.
- Create circular paths or enclosed outdoor gardens that will facilitate safe wandering.
- Put hedges or fence around patio or yard.
- Create garden walls so the person can be outside safely.
- Surround the yard with protective fencing.
- Camouflage gates or other exits.
- Provide opportunities for meaningful activity such as a swing or safe place to garden.

The Inside Environment

- Ensure that house is well lit.
- Assess the inside environment for cues for wandering, such as coats, hats, or umbrellas hung near the exit doors.
- Consider camouflage techniques such as covering the door with a curtain or screen. This blocks the easy view of exit doors.
- Install multistep or complex door fasteners.
- Use a dead bolt keeping the key handy for emergencies.
- Use a safety latch that prevents the person with Alzheimer's from opening the door.
- Place door locks out of the normal line of vision, either very high or very low.
- Create a "barrier" by applying a double line of brightly colored tape to the floor.
- Set up a safe area in the home where the person can wander at night.
- Use night-lights.
- Install gates at stairwells.
- Install electronic buzzers, chimes, bells, or other types of alarms at exits.
- Use childproof doorknob covers.
- Install monitor system.
- Use guards or locks on windows.
- Hide doorknobs behind cloth panels.
- Move doorknobs and locks from conventional locations.
- Place a black door mat in front of the exit door—the person with dementia might see it as a hole and will not step over it due to the visual spatial problems that accompany the disease.
- Put a stop sign on the door.
- Place police tape across the door.
- Install a battery-operated intercom or monitoring system that will allow the caregiver to hear what the person is doing in other rooms.
- Use a pressure-sensitive mat so that if the person gets of bed, the caregiver will know it.
- Provide 24-hour supervision, as "These methods are not foolproof and do not replace careful supervision" (Algase, 1992, p. 32).

Community strategies

- Register the person with dementia in the national Safe Return program through your local Alzheimer's Association chapter. Assistance from

Safe Return is available 24 hours a day by calling 1-800-572-1122 whenever someone with dementia wanders away from home or a facility, or is found in the community, lost and confused. There is a nominal, one-time registration fee, currently $40, and scholarship aid is available from the Alzheimer's Association and from some state agencies (for more on Safe Return, see chapter 5).

- Inform the neighbors of the situation.
- Let the local police know of the situation.
- Keep an item of the patient's clothing in a sealed plastic bag in the event that it is needed by a search and rescue canine unit.
- Make sure all of the caregivers involved in the care of the person are aware of the person's propensity to wander.

Stimulation strategies

- Encourage movement and exercise in safe areas. Safe areas are secured areas. Make exercise a shared experience as part of a daily routine. Exercise helps to reduce anxiety and restlessness; supervised walking or "walking with a buddy" is highly recommended.
- Involve the person in productive daily activities such as folding laundry or preparing dinner.
- Interventions such as music (or pet) therapy help keep the person engaged.
- Increase activity during the day so that the person may sleep better at night.
- Enroll the person in an adult day health program (adult day care). By going to the day care, the person with dementia is kept active and awake during the day.
- Provide activity that is appropriate to the functioning level of the person based on past interests or work.
- Provide a rocking chair or other chair that swivels or rocks; rocking may help to relieve restlessness.

Monitoring strategies

- Provide opportunities for supervised walking. Find or hire someone to walk with the person with Alzheimer's—a "walking buddy."
- Use redirection: guide or distract the person from hallways and doors.
- Assure the person with dementia who is insistent that he does not have to go to a specific place (e.g., work, home, to see his mother) at this

time. Use diversionary strategies such as offering food or another activity. Do not tell the person that he no longer works or that his mother has died—these types of statements serve only to elicit emotions of loss, but rather use what have been referred to as "therapeutic fiblets," e.g., "You're on vacation," or "Your mother is not home right now." These strategies are part of a concept of care called habilitation therapy. (For more on this approach see Raia & Koenig-Coste, 1996).

- Remind the person that you know how to find him/her and that he/she is in the right place. Providing reassurance is the best strategy for caring for an individual with dementia.
- Reassure the person who may feel lost, abandoned, or disoriented.

Finally, the Alzheimer's Association, Massachusetts Chapter (2001) in its *Family Care Guide* provides the following helpful advice to caregivers to increase their ability to understand and cope with the issues associated with wandering and driving.

Driving Strategies

Alzheimer's disease, in its earliest stages, shortens attention span and affects judgment, reaction time, and visual-spatial abilities. One study found that 44% of newly diagnosed patients who still drove a car routinely got lost. A study of older drivers found that people with Alzheimer's were 19 times more likely to be involved in a crash than those without the disease. Another examined the brains of elderly drivers killed in crashes and found that one third showed clear evidence of early Alzheimer's. There is no argument that at some point, people with the disease will be unable to drive safely. Driving is an issue that needs to be addressed sensitively—and early—in the disease process.

Guidelines of the American Psychiatric Association urge physicians to encourage even their mildly impaired dementia patients to stop driving. The American Academy of Neurology, recognizing that people with early Alzheimer's are at an increased risk of car crashes, has issued guidelines to help doctors determine when patients should stop driving. In discussing the driving issue, patients, caregivers and doctors should also know that the ethical guidelines of the American Medical Association make public safety a priority over patient confidentiality, allowing physicians to notify their state's Department of Motor Vehicles when a patient's diagnosis makes him or her unsafe to drive.

Many people with Alzheimer's disease recognize that they are losing their ability to drive safely. With the support of family and professional caregivers, they voluntarily stop. Others continue to drive because they fear losing their sense of independence and competence. Some, because of the disease, just cannot recognize the danger they pose to themselves and others. Caregivers can meet strong resistance to giving up the keys.

- Be careful not to overwhelm the cognitively-impaired individual with demands that he stop driving at a time when he may still be reeling, emotionally, from news of his diagnosis.
- Be just as careful not to let yourself become the focus of his anger at the idea that he stop driving.
- At the time of diagnosis, the doctor should always ask if the patient still drives. In explaining the diagnosis, the doctor can gently point out the problem. If the doctor does not ask, then the individual receiving the diagnosis or a family member should ask the doctor directly.
- Ask the doctor to write a note or prescription that specifically says she is not to drive.
- After the visit, remind the patient that her doctor said she should no longer drive.
- Have someone else in whom the patient may have a special trust reinforce the no-driving message.
- Ask your family's attorney or insurance agent to reinforce that message by explaining the potential for liability.
- Have the patient's driving skills assessed through a driving fitness evaluation program. The local Alzheimer's Association, state Department of Motor Vehicles or AARP will know of these programs. They should include provisions for counseling, periodic retesting, and include a road test along with other evaluations.
- Offer to drive. Get backup driving help from family members or volunteers.
- When practical, use home delivery services rather than having the patient drive to shops.
- Check local resources and agencies such as your town's Council on Aging or Senior Center for alternative, supervised transportation when you or your backup driver cannot transport the patient.

It is important that all of the patient's caregivers agree on their approach to this issue. If someone you care about has Alzheimer's disease, is still driving, and others in the family do not agree that he should give up the keys, ask them these questions:

- Would you be comfortable with your young child or grandchild riding in the same car?
- Would you be comfortable with your young child or grandchild stepping out into a pedestrian crosswalk in front of the car?

This is a tough issue—not addressing it does not make it go away and could result in a catastrophic consequence for the individual or innocent bystanders.

Some patients who drive will claim that they don't drive very far from home, drive slowly, or use only familiar routes. While these claims appear reassuring, most crashes occur at lower speeds, at intersections, and near home. Some caregivers act as "copilots" for their spouses with Alzheimer's who drive. This is a risky and unreliable fix, since it cannot repair the central problem of the driver's progressively declining memory, reaction time, and judgment.

Different strategies may work for different patients who should not drive:

- Involve the patient's doctor in a family conference to discuss a strategy.
- Be honest with the patient. Tell him that he has a problem with his memory and that it is not safe for him to drive.
- Seeing the car is a visual cue to use it. Remove it, garage it, or park it out of sight with a neighbor or friend.
- Car keys are another visual cue. Keep the car locked and control access to the keys.
- Have a mechanic install a "kill switch" that in the off position will prevent the car from starting. Some stores sell car batteries with an "off" switch. If necessary, disconnect the battery, distributor cap, or starter wire to make the car inoperable.
- When he asks where it is, tell him the car is not working, is in the shop, or that a relative borrowed it.
- Some charities accept older cars as donations. If the patient has a favorite charity, tell him that it was his decision to donate it after the doctor suggested he stop driving.
- When he talks about wanting the car, distract or redirect him by changing the subject, telling him you're not ready to go yet, or that he should eat before leaving.
- If these various strategies are just not working and the patient continues to drive in an unsafe way, anyone caring for or interacting with him, including police, can notify the state Department of Motor Vehicles (usually through its medical affairs unit) that they believe his driving poses a risk to himself or others. The DMV can retest the patient.

A note and a caution about technological devices in cars:

- Satellite-based Global Positioning System navigation devices come installed in some luxury cars, and can be purchased for others. These require that the driver be ready and able to use them. For a patient with a serious memory impairment who is lost, manipulating this device may be a problem.
- Antitheft devices such as Lojack are also available for cars, but they are designed for use when a car is stolen, not when the driver is lost.
- None of these devices will prevent unsafe driving.

Be firm, but avoid arguments about driving. Focus on other activities that the person with Alzheimer's can enjoy and still do successfully. (For more on driving and dementia see *Tips for Balancing Independence and Safety, Warning Signs Worksheet* or *Agreement With Family About Driving* available at www.thehartford.com)

CHAPTER 8

The Facility: Recommendations for Long-Term Care and Assisted Living Residences

In the following pages, we make recommendations and suggest strategies to help staff and management of long-term care facilities and assisted living residences create a safe environment related to wandering.

We focus on recommended techniques to help facilities cope with wandering and improve the safety of the environment in this chapter for three important reasons:

1. Nearly half of all those in long-term care settings have some form of dementia and thus are at risk for wandering.
2. Wandering episodes and attempts often result in serious consequences such as injury, hospitalization, or even death.
3. There are many safeguards that can be taken to minimize wandering episodes, and there are effective practices for dealing with situations when the person is in fact missing.

Many Nursing Home and Assisted Living Residents Are at Risk for Wandering

While the literature asserts that wandering is widespread among people with dementia living in the community, the research also suggests that it is common among those living in long-term care facilities, at least half of whom are estimated to have some form of cognitive impairment such as Alzheimer's disease (Kennedy, 1993).

In fact, as detailed in chapter 2 many studies of wandering have focused their investigations of this behavior on people living in nursing homes or assisted living residences. The wandering problem has been estimated to range from 11% (Hiatt, 1985) to 24% (Hoffman, Platt, & Barry, 1987). Burnside (1981) reports that approximately 20% of the staff in long-term care facilities are aware of at least one incident resulting in the serious injury or death of a wanderer, and a survey of administrators, directors of nursing, and nursing personnel revealed that 41% believed that wandering was the leading behavioral problem while at least 80% of the nursing directors mentioned wandering as a problem in general (Wickersty, 1986).

Kennedy (1993) estimates that each week at least one resident of this country's nursing home facilities will wander off the premises and die. A study of insurance claims against nursing homes reveals the following relevant points: 1) 70% of elopement claims involve the death of a resident; 2) 45% of elopements occurred within the first 48 hours of admission; and, 3) 80% of elopements involved chronic or repeat wanderers (Rodriguez, 1993).

Attempts at wandering are also a problem in institutions. Gaffney (1986) found that over a 15-hour period, 28 wanderers attempted to leave a nursing home unit 457 times and attempted to use an exit 274 times.

When considering a common problem behavior such as wandering, it is important to understand its economic impact as well as its stressful and dangerous nature. There is often a large cost associated with the recovery of those who have wandered and become lost. Such costs are accrued "in terms of lost time for nursing home staff and often the public safety costs of police, fire, and rescue units searching for these individuals" (Coombs, 1994, p. 204).

Several authors offer details about such costs with Butler and Barnett (1991) citing the expense of a search effort as averaging about $2500 per episode. Similarly, Kennedy (1993) reports that "nonproductive man hours spent in checking the whereabouts of wanderers average $2500 per patient per year. Thus, the worker costs to a home with ten wandering patients would be about $25,000 a year" (p. 172). We would also note that search and rescue costs can quickly mushroom, and may often be underreported.

Before turning to specific suggestions for creating a safe environment and coping with wandering in the facility, we would reiterate that people with dementia should be presumed at high risk for wandering due to their cognitive deficits and unpredictable behavior (Coltharp, Richie, & Kaas, 1996; Flaherty & Raia, 1994). Any interventions or management strategies must also take this important fact into account.

Moreover, in the past, interventions in nursing home facilities mainly involved the use of physical and chemical restraints. Algase (1992) reports that "until the passage of the Nursing Home Reform Act, part of OBRA 1987, the 11 to 39% of nursing home residents who wander were almost sure to experience restraint" (p. 28). While the Omnibus Budget Reconciliation Act of 1987 (OBRA) mandates that neither physical nor chemical restraints can be used to treat wandering in nursing home residents, it is also important to note that there are numerous problems with each of these methods of restraint.

Physical restraints often result in serious injuries (King & Mallet, 1991) and increased agitation (Werner, Cohen-Mansfield, Braun, & Marx, 1989). More specifically, Souren and colleagues argue that "physical restraint does not relieve the existing anxiety and agitation and often leads to more disruptive behaviors, such as screaming and aggression. Restraint also promotes a premature loss of ambulation, with the risk of contracture formation in large joints (Souren, Franssen, & Reisberg, 1995).

Chemical restraints, on the other hand, cause serious side effects (King & Mallet, 1991). Others point out that "intervention with psychoactive medication can alleviate agitation, but it may further decrease cognitive abilities and is often not effective in stopping wandering" (McCarten, Kovera, Maddox, & Cleary, 1995).

In light of the evidence on the complications and dangers of physical and chemical restraints, nursing homes and other facilities must focus on safer and more effective interventions that accommodate the behavior rather than eliminate it. "An appropriately designed and implemented environment and treatment program should strive to eliminate almost any need for physical or chemical restraints. When restraints are the only appropriate alternative, written policies and procedures must exist that comply with legislative and statutory regulations for their use. These guidelines should include education and training requirements for staff, residents, and families; procedures to obtain informed consent; consistent monitoring; documentation of the rationale for and continued use of restraints; regular observation and reporting to ensure that guidelines are followed; and periodic reviews of policies and procedures" (Karcher, 1993).

Not every safety strategy will work for every facility. For example, some strategies apply to those facilities being newly designed while others are appropriate for existing facilities. Furthermore, assisted living facilities will require a different overall approach than many nursing home settings. While many of the strategies suggested in the following pages will be effective and possible to implement in both nursing homes and assisted living residences, some simply will not be feasible in the assisted living facility. Foltz-Gray

(1997) talks about the intricacies involved stating that "for the administrator and staff of any assisted living facility, these behaviors, often loosely identified as 'wandering,' complicate what used to be a simple notion: that residents in an assisted living facility can live independently and privately, and with less intense care than a nursing home provides . . . Managing the wandering of those residents without compromising the safety, dignity, and autonomy of all residents isn't easy" (p. 54).

In assisted living facilities, unlike nursing homes, there are no locked hallways, the population is not as physically frail or ill, the residents need more opportunities for exercise and activities due to the fact that they are more physically healthy, and there is not as much of an emphasis on clinical care. While these characteristics do pose unique challenges, they must be addressed. Fifty percent of the assisted living facility residents having Alzheimer's disease or other form of dementia (Foltz-Gray, 1997), wandering and the propensity to wander and get lost are serious problems. Some assisted living facilities simply will not accept residents who wander, in the belief that all residents should have an environment where they can come and go as they please. Also, many are just not equipped or staffed to deal with this problem.

It is important to remember that to varying degrees, the challenge in both settings is to maintain safety in the least restrictive environment and to use interventions that help promote independence and self-determination.

Not every intervention will work for every resident. Wandering is not a simple behavior and those who are likely to wander are not a homogenous group. In the following pages, we offer an array of safety techniques for dealing with the problem of wandering. We encourage facilities to begin by conducting necessary assessments, which are described in greater detail later in this chapter, and then to try different strategies and find the ones that work and are most effective for them and the populations they serve. It is highly recommended that long-term care residences have several interventions in place on an ongoing basis—if one technique fails, there are other safeguards in place. Interventions must be multifaceted and geared to the specific needs of the individual resident.

Recommended Management Strategies

We begin by recommending precautions aimed at preventing unsafe wandering from happening. We then turn to measures that should be taken when wandering has already occurred and the person with dementia is lost.

Strategies to protect individuals and long-term care facilities from the risks associated with wandering can be grouped as follows: 1) *environmental management strategies* for both the interior and exterior. This would include design and layout features as well as the use of assistive devices and techniques such as alarms, camouflage, and other exit control techniques; 2) *formal strategies* such as assessments at the individual and facility levels, developing a lost person plan, conducting appropriate staff training, and other organizational policies such as registering the person with Safe Return; 3) *stimulation strategies* such as providing increased activity, chores, and stimulation during the day, as well as eliminating negative stimulation and creating a calm environment; 4) *visual cues* such as using "stop" signs; and 5) *monitoring strategies* including walking with, following, or shadowing the person.

Environmental management strategies

Managing the environment includes considering both the outside surroundings as well as the interior of the facility and should begin with a careful assessment of the two environments followed by the implementation of appropriate interventions. Thomas (1995) recommends "a useful evaluation tool developed by Zeisel, Hyde, & Levkoff (1994) which assesses several environmental factors critical to the functional abilities of people with dementia. Several factors have special importance when assessing the environment for the continuous wanderer (i.e., exit control, wandering paths, autonomy support, and sensory comprehension)" (p. 39). These are discussed in more detail in chapter 6. The goal is to develop areas indoors and outdoors where people can explore and wander safely and independently.

The Outside Environment

- Review the environment in and around the facility for possible hazards—swimming pools, dense foliage, tunnels, steep stairways, high balconies, and roadways where traffic tends to be heavy—and limit access to potentially dangerous areas.
- Consider approaches to enhance safe exercise in secured areas. Create circular paths or enclosed outdoor gardens that will facilitate outdoor freedom. The circular or continuous layout will help minimize decision points for residents.
- Create places to sit that have interesting views. Taft and colleagues (1993) recommend "walkways with continuous loops where activity alcoves and rest areas allow for wandering without getting lost. The

rest areas divert the clients' attention away from exhaustive repetitious wandering and invite the client to engage in other activities" (p. 2).

- Provide opportunities for meaningful activity such as a swing, bench, or safe planter.
- Camouflage gates or other exits.

The Inside Environment

- Assess the inside environment for cues for wandering. Exit Control—doors, door handles, and security devices should be minimally visible. Install door alarms, video surveillance, and electronic tracking devices. Recent advances have made such systems and devices more user-friendly for staff and residents. When considering an alarm system, select one that is pleasant sounding and subdued so as not to frighten residents. Brawley (1997) notes that bells and alarms to alert staff that a resident is trying to open a door may prevent a resident from leaving a safe environment, but they can also disrupt that environment and the noise they create can cause other problems, including heightened anxiety and catastrophic reactions. A fuller discussion of exit control systems and the use of technology for managing wandering is in chapter 5 of this book. It is important to note that technology should be used to enhance the actions of well-trained staff and not substitute for such training.
- Consider camouflage techniques such as covering the door with a curtain or screen, painting exit doors the same color as the walls, or concealment of the doorknob behind a cloth panel. Because patients do not always understand why they cannot enter an area, camouflage can be the most effective means of control (Stehman, et al., 1996).
- Provide adequately illuminated walkways without obstacles and with recognizable points of reference. Thomas (1995) notes that "having adequate glare-free lighting along with minimizing environmental hazards should be included when designing a therapeutic milieu for the continuous wanderer" (p. 39). Special lighting and windows serve to eliminate shadow, disorientation, and glare.
- Create a homelike environment—refer to the large meeting room as the living room instead of the day room or lounge. When adapting existing structures or facilities, large activity rooms and dining areas can be overstimulating. Staff could change the environment by using partitions or even furniture to divide the large space into two or more self-contained areas.

Formal strategies

Formal strategies such as conducting facility and individual level assessments, developing a missing person plan, conducting appropriate staff training, and other organizational policies such as registering the person with Safe Return are important components in dealing with the problem behavior of wandering and getting lost. Davis (1996) concurs, stating that an effective program "should develop an assessment protocol for residents, perform a facility risk assessment, install devices as needed, and train and evaluate staff continuously" (p. 34).

Following the formal strategies outlined below provides a facility with one of the most critical characteristics needed to serve persons with Alzheimer's disease and related dementias—being prepared.

Assessments

Assessment of the facility/environment

- Decide if the facility is prepared to care for the wanderer or cannot accept those who are at high risk for wandering.
- Conduct a risk assessment of both the inside and outside environments. Also, identify any cues for wandering such as items that may trigger the desire to go out—coatrack, umbrella, purse.

Assessment of individual residents

- What is learned in the assessment can then be used to tailor effective interventions.
- An assessment includes looking at the possible reasons for wandering. Assess frequency, timing, and length of wandering episodes. Were there any precursors such as hunger, cold, or wanting to go home? Attempts to identify the causative factors are essential to the development of an individualized care plan.
- Questions are a crucial part of an assessment:

    1. Did anything happen just before the episode that could have caused it?
    2. Is there a time pattern?
    3. Is the person looking for activity or exercise?
    4. Does the person appear to have a goal?

5. Is the person on any medications that might cause restlessness?
6. Is there a physical complaint that is the basis of the wandering? (Looking for the bathroom, feeling cold or hungry, for example)

- Thomas (1995) suggests that "discussing the history of the wanderer with the family is a critical component of the assessment" (p. 39). An assessment should include information from the patients as well as their family caregivers.
- Resident service plans should address the resident's risk of wandering, when applicable, and goals and approaches should be formulated.
- Sutor, Rummans, and Smith (2001) demonstrate how an individual assessment can help facilities tailor the most effective interventions. In their article on suggested strategies for management of behavior problems, they suggest the following (p. 544):

TABLE 8.1 Suggested Strategies for Management of Behavior Problems

Behavior	Potential Cause or Antecedent	Management Strategy
Wandering	Stress—noise, clutter, crowding	Reduce excessive stimulation
	Lost—looking for someone or something familiar	Provide familiar objects, signs, pictures; offer to help; reassure
	Restless—bored, no stimuli	Provide meaningful activity
	Medication side effect	Monitor, reduce, or discontinue medication
	Lifelong pattern of being active	Provide safe area to move about
	Needing to use the toilet	Institute toileting schedule; place signs or pictures on bathroom door
	Environmental stimuli—exit signs, people leaving	Remove or camouflage environmental stimuli; provide identification or alarm bracelets

Staff Training and Personnel Issues

Facilities should have an optimal staff to resident ratio of 1:5; or an adequate staffing ratio of 1:6 or 1:7 (Kennedy, 1993). Such staffing ratios allow for the careful supervision that is needed to manage wandering and getting lost. It is important to note that there are no failproof methods and careful supervision is always warranted.

Staff should be:

- Trained in ways of approaching the wanderer
  Never confront or argue when approaching.
  Foster trust through eye contact and nonthreatening interaction.
  Avoid catastrophic reactions.
  Communicate reassurance in voice and manner.
- Trained to respond with creativity and acceptance, not in punitive and controlling ways.
- Trained to recognize the importance of a person's need to move—design the environment to allow for safe mobility.
- Educated about all interventions including alarm systems.
- Trained on wandering risk.
- Assigned responsibility for regular checks.
- Accountable for each resident's whereabouts on the shift change report.
- Trained to communicate with families. Communication and understanding are important to successful management.
- Aware of each resident's propensity to wander. Staff should also be trained to alert and instruct visitors and volunteers regarding wandering behavior alarm systems and appropriate responses.

A change in interventions is not necessarily accompanied by a change in staff attitudes or beliefs about wandering behavior and its problems. The knowledge has to be incorporated into the mainstream of a facility.

Enroll residents with dementia in Safe Return, use identification

Ensure that residents are wearing some form of identification. Employ a range of identification systems including sewing identification into the person's clothing. Facilities should participate in a safety/identification program. The Safe Return program, operated by the Alzheimer's Association in cooperation with the U.S. Justice Department, is a nationwide system designed to help identify, locate, and return to safety individuals who are memory impaired due to Alzheimer's disease or a related disorder (see chapter 5 for more on this program) (Alzheimer's Disease and Related Disorders Association, 1996).

Stimulation and orienting strategies

Provide Positive Stimulation

- Allow for safe exercise. An example of a formal program that provides such an opportunity is a nursing home walking program staffed by volunteers in a 450-bed geriatric facility in New York State. Supervised by clinical staff, volunteers complete a 4-hour training and orientation program. A psychiatric nurse clinical specialist works with the volunteers each evening during the first 2 weeks of the program (Holmberg, 1997).
- Provide a consistent daily schedule as well as consistency in caregivers.
- Provide opportunities for sensory stimulation—examples include soft, textured wall hangings; baseball cards; t-shirts to fold; buttons.
- Thomas (1995) suggests that "designing an interesting environment through tactile and sensory cues could potentially redirect the continuous wanderer to stop his/her motion and perhaps be compelled to sit" (p. 39). Along these same lines, Gaffney (1986) recommends that staff "develop environmental cues such as sensory tables, tactile boards and 'activity barrels,' all of which use familiar items to attract the wanderer's attention. Integral to the success of using familiar props is the comprehensive assessment of the wanderer's previous lifestyle, likes and dislikes, meaningful activities and roles" (pp. 94–96).
- Alleviate boredom through creative programming—dance groups, music, etc.
- Schedule outings and physically active games.
- Provide opportunities for exercise particularly when people are waiting for a meal or activity. Exercise might also include singing, rhythmic movements, dancing, etc.
- Provide rocking chairs or other chairs that swivel or rock; rocking may help to relieve restlessness.

Eliminate Negative Stimulation

- Minimize inappropriate stimuli or stimulation that seems to trigger the problem behavior.
- Reduce amounts of noise and confusion in the environment.

- Offer structure with flexibility. The predictable organization of person, time, and place reduces disorientation and anxiety.
- Specifically, Thomas (1995) suggests that "efforts should be made to create an atmosphere that is calm and relaxed by eliminating disturbing sounds such as the clanging of carts, loud chatter, voices on the intercom, TVs and radios" (p. 39).

Orienting strategies

- Provide way-finding cues, such as clear paths to destinations with arrows or lines on the floor, or physical landmarks such as signs and pictures. While these help with the problem of wandering, they also help residents to maintain independence.
- Orient residents using personal mementos as landmarks.
- Reinforce location of bathrooms and other public areas by having rooms clearly labeled, painted bright colors, or marked with icons, lights, or awnings.

Visual Cues and Barriers

Visual cues and barriers capitalize on the cognitive deficits and visual agnosia present in those with Alzheimer's disease or related disorders.

- Try a yellow strip of plastic (symbolizing caution) that is velcroed across doors to prevent residents from exiting. The strip is easy to get through in case of emergency and allows patients to keep their doors open to see and hear what is happening inside or outside their room.
- A large NO! or a stop sign on doors may discourage residents from entering or exiting.
- Try a mini blind concealing the view of the door, and a cloth panel concealing the doorknob and panic bar of the door (Dickinson, McLain-Kark, & Marshall-Baker, 1995).
- Place a black doormat in front of the exit door—the person with dementia might see it as a hole and will not step over it due to the visual spatial problems that accompany the disease. Masking tape placed in grids on the floor in front of the door may also prove effective.

Monitoring strategies

- It is important to note that 45% of elopements occur within the first 48 hours of admission (Rodriguez, 1993). The adjustment of moving to a new and unfamiliar place is difficult and special precautions should be taken during the first few days of a resident's move into a facility. It may be possible for a family member to spend most of the first few days with the patient. Careful supervision by facility staff is key during this transitional period.

- Provide opportunities for supervised walking. Staff or volunteers (as was described earlier in this chapter) could walk with the person with Alzheimer's—each resident could be assigned a "walking buddy."
- Have someone go for a walk outdoors with the person who is determined to "go home." Eventually the person may tire or become distracted.
- Use redirection: guide or distract the person from hallways, doors. Distracting with food, drink, or activity might be helpful.
- Assure the person with dementia that they do not have to go to a specific place (work, to see their mother) at this time; use of the term "later" may help. Do not tell the person that they no longer work or that their mother has died—these types of statements serve only to elicit emotions of loss.
- If wandering behavior occurs in the evening and person is determined to "go home" for example, try suggesting that the person spend the night since it is late, and go home in the morning.
- Remind the person that you know how to find him and that he is in the right place. Providing reassurance and validation is the best strategy for caring for an individual with dementia.
- Reassure the person who may feel lost, abandoned, or disoriented.
- Install an intercom or monitoring system that will allow staff to hear what the person is doing in other rooms.
- Use a pressure-sensitive mat so that if the person gets out of bed, staff will know it.
- Provide 24-hour supervision.

When Wandering Has Occurred and a Resident Is Lost or Missing

It is important to develop and implement a lost person plan. Have a written plan for risk management and a plan of action in place in case someone wanders away from the facility.

The following Missing Resident Protocol is currently in place in facilities being operated by a national provider, and serves as a model example of steps to take when a resident is missing or lost.

❐ The staff person who is unable to locate a resident should immediately notify the Executive Director or designee of the facility.

❐ The Executive Director or designee should alert all staff of the missing resident and give a description of the resident and the last time and place the resident was seen.

❐ The Executive Director or designee should assign each employee a specific area to search. These areas must includes storage areas, halls, kitchen, activity area, lounges, common areas, and stairways. It is important to open all closets and doors to make sure the resident is not hiding, injured, or asleep.

❐ If the resident is still not located, the Executive Director or designee should assign employees to search the facility grounds, including parked cars, nearby bus stops, or other pick-up points.

If the above steps have been completed and the resident has still not been located, the Executive Director or designee should take the following steps:

❐ notify all management and staff of the facility

❐ notify the family member(s) and/or other responsible parties indicated in the resident's file. Alert them to the fact that the person is missing and describe the steps that have been taken to locate the resident. Ask the family members and/or other parties whether they are aware of the resident's location. Ask for any possible places the resident would likely visit, such as former residences and other family or friends' residences.

❐ Notify the Police Department.

❐ give a complete description of the resident to give the police, including the following information:

a. Name
b. Sex
c. Race
d. Age
e. Height
f. Weight
g. Hair color
h. Eye color
i. Clothing worn when last seen
j. Time discovered missing
k. Physical and mental capacities and limitation such as mobility,

mental state, and physical limitations

l. A recent photo of resident should be supplied

m. The resident's history of wandering or leaving the facility, including prior places resident was found

n. Place of residence outside the community and place of residence of any close family or friend or other location where the resident might go

o. All steps undertaken to locate the resident

- ❒ Follow the instructions of the officer in charge.
- ❒ If there is a possibility that the resident may have left the area, you may need to consider notifying the Sheriff's Department or State Patrol. Consult with the Police Department regarding other agencies to contact.
- ❒ If the resident is registered with the Alzheimer's Association Safe Return program, the national emergency number should be called: 1-800-572-1122.
- ❒ Be prepared to give the resident's Safe Return registration identification number.
- ❒ If it is deemed appropriate, either because of the length of time the resident has been missing or the jeopardy in which the resident may be placed in by virtue of being away from the facility, consideration should be given to contacting various news media (radio, TV, newspaper, etc.).
- ❒ The Executive Director should contact the Vice President of Operations for consent prior to calling any news media.
- ❒ Only the Vice President of Operations, Executive Director or designee should contact the news media. No other facility employee should give out any information.
- ❒ Any inquiry by newspaper, telephone, or radio concerning a missing resident should be referred to the Executive Director. No other employee should give out any information.
- ❒ Refer to your facility's Public Relations policy.

After the resident has been found, the following steps should be taken:

- ❒ Assess the resident's physical condition. If there appears to be any change in the physical or mental status, immediately notify the attending physician.
- ❒ Promptly notify everyone involved in the search effort.

- ❐ Notify the family member or responsible party.
- ❐ Document, in the resident's medical record, the details of the event including the following information:

  a. Condition of the resident prior to incident
  b. Time resident was discovered missing
  c. Last place the resident was seen
  d. *Complete* description of the search effort, including notification of facility staff, authorities, family, etc.
  e. Time the resident was found
  f. Place the resident was found
  g. Findings regarding the resident's physical and mental status upon return to the facility
  h. Details regarding the manner in which the event occurred
  i. Document notification of physician and family, as well as state agencies and police if applicable
  j. Any information that would prevent a recurrence

- ❐ Meet with facility search team members to reassess and critique the security and the search procedure.
- ❐ Complete an event report for the facility file. The event form should not be kept in the resident's health record.
- ❐ Review report at any safety committee meeting.

CHAPTER 9

The Community: Recommendations for Elder Care and Acute Care Providers

Elder Care Providers

All agencies and facilities that provide services to elders should take precautions against unsafe wandering. The U.S. Congress, Office of Technology Assessment (1990) and the Alzheimer's Association (1997) have defined agencies that serve elders as dementia-specific, dementia-capable, or dementia-friendly. Dementia-specific agencies are those that serve individuals with Alzheimer's disease or a related disorder exclusively. Dementia-capable agencies are those that have staff who are trained in dementia care, but also serve elders who are not cognitively impaired. Dementia-friendly agencies are agencies that serve all elders but do not have staff members that are specifically trained in dementia care.

Just because a facility is not "dementia-specific" does not mean that individuals with dementia will not utilize the programs available and services provided by that facility. Social day care, adult day health, assisted living, councils on aging/senior centers, and religious and civic organizations that run programs for elders, all would benefit by heightened awareness of the likelihood of wandering by individuals with cognitive impairments who may utilize their programs. Moreover, agency staff can be proactive in alerting individuals and family members to the ten warning signs of dementia and encourage diagnostic screening when concerns are raised. If dementia is suspected, then the potential for wandering should be assumed. Thus, the first recommendation to elder care providers is to be familiar with the warning signs of Alzheimer's disease.

The ten warning signs underscore that Alzheimer's disease is not just memory loss. People with Alzheimer's disease experience a decline in cognitive abilities, such as thinking and understanding, and changes in behavior. The Alzheimer's Association has developed a list of warning signs that include common symptoms of Alzheimer's disease (some also apply to other dementias). If an elder care worker notices several of these symptoms, that worker should recommend to the individual or a family member that a physician should be seen for a complete examination. The ten warning signs listed below have been modified slightly to reflect elder care settings (adapted from Alzheimer's Association, 2001).

The ten warning signs

1. **Memory loss that affects job, volunteer, or daily skills.** It is normal to occasionally forget an assignment, deadline, or colleague's name, but frequent forgetfulness or unexplainable confusion at home, in the workplace, or elder care setting may signal that something is wrong.
2. **Difficulty performing familiar tasks.** Busy people get distracted from time to time. For example, you might leave something on the stove too long or not remember to serve part of a meal. People with Alzheimer's might prepare a meal and not only forget to serve it but also forget they made it.
3. **Problems with language.** Everyone has trouble finding the right word sometimes, but a person with Alzheimer's disease may forget simple words or substitute inappropriate words, making his or her sentences difficult to understand.
4. **Disorientation to time and place.** It is normal to momentarily forget the day of the week or what you need from the store. But people with Alzheimer's disease can become lost on their own street, not knowing where they are, how they got there, or how to get back home.
5. **Poor or decreased judgment.** Choosing not to bring a sweater or coat along on a chilly night is a common mistake. A person with Alzheimer's, however, may dress inappropriately in more noticeable ways, wearing a bathrobe to the store or several blouses on a hot day.
6. **Problems with abstract thinking.** Balancing a checkbook can be challenging for many people, but for someone with Alzheimer's, recognizing numbers or performing basic calculations may be impossible.

7. **Misplacing things.** Everyone temporarily misplaces a wallet or keys from time to time. A person with Alzheimer's disease may put these and other items in inappropriate places—such as an iron in the freezer or a wristwatch in the sugar bowl—and then not recall how they got there. In addition, a person with Alzheimer's may look at the keys and not know their purpose.
8. **Changes in mood or behavior.** Everyone experiences a broad range of emotions—it is part of being human. People with Alzheimer's tend to exhibit more rapid mood swings for no apparent reason.
9. **Changes in personality.** Personalities may change somewhat as people age. But a person with Alzheimer's can change dramatically, either suddenly or over a period of time. Someone who is generally easygoing may become angry, suspicious, or fearful.
10. **Loss of initiative.** It is normal to tire of housework, business activities, or social obligations, but most people retain or eventually regain their interest. The person with Alzheimer's disease may remain uninterested and uninvolved in many or all of his/her usual pursuits.

Environmental audit

The next recommendation, after elder care agencies are familiar with the warning signs of dementia, is for the agencies to conduct an environmental "audit" of their indoor and outdoor physical space. Our feeling is that modifications that are done to respond to the needs of cognitively impaired elders will, for the most part, improve environments for the general population of elders as well. Referring back to the criteria defined in chapter 6, how does the facility rate on exit control, wandering paths, and outdoor space?

Exit control

- Exit doors should be nonobtrusive so cognitively impaired elders will not be attracted to them.
- Signals or other control devices with few delays in warning should be in place so that staff is immediately aware in the event that an elopement takes place.
- Exit doors located off of a common room or on the side of or alcove off a main hallway are less likely to visibly cue cognitively impaired elders.
- Exit doors should have few signs, windows, or visible hardware.
- The area on the other side of an exit door should be safe in case a cognitively impaired elder does elope.

Wandering paths

- Corridors and other pathways in the facility provide cognitively impaired elders with understandable visual cues and interesting events that support therapeutic walking.
- A sign is an overt cue indicating where to go (bathroom) or how to behave (no smoking). A less overt cue might be a change in floor covering helping residents to sense the difference between a hallway and an activity room.
- The more elements of interest along a pathway (views, artwork, benches), the more interesting the path is for cognitively impaired elders.
- A continuous path with turning potential and places along the path that provide purposeful destinations is the most desirable goal.

Outdoor space

- Outdoor space is accessible immediately adjacent to the elder care agency and secure enough for cognitively impaired elders to come and go independently.
- The outdoor space has physical elements that support cognitively impaired elders to function effectively outdoors.
- Outdoor space is on the same level as staff offices and allows for easy surveillance by staff and enables cognitively impaired elders to use the space at their own discretion.
- The outdoor space has high enclosures and is locked. The likelihood of serious consequences from eloping from the outdoor space is minimal.
- The outdoor space is dedicated for use with cognitively impaired elders.

Policies and protocols

Policies and protocols should be in place for responding to a wandering episode. Such protocols should include registering cognitively impaired elders in Safe Return as part of the initial intake or assessment for program or services. A current photograph of the elder should also be provided to the agency upon initial intake. Protocols should follow the recommendations provided by Safe Return:

Five Steps to Take Immediately When a Memory Impaired Person Has Wandered Off

1. **Have staff search** the vicinity in the first 15 minutes. Do it immediately. Be thorough.

2. Then **notify local police**. Call them right away. Do not wait. If elder has not been registered in Safe Return, make sure you have a recent photograph available to assist police.
3. Next, **call 1-800-572-1122**. Report the missing elder to the national alert operator. Say if the missing elder is wearing identification. Confirm that you completed steps 1 and 2 above.
4. **Call** a family member of the elder or designated care provider.
5. **Stay by the phone.** You or someone else must be available to assist in the safe return of the missing patient. Keep all other incoming and outgoing calls as brief as possible. Stay calm and focused.

Training

- Dementia care training should be provided to all staff members from custodial to administration.
- Training should include initial orientation, in-service training, and the opportunities for professional growth and development such as attending off-site workshops, conferences, and academic classes. In addition to staff, volunteers should also receive dementia care training. The local chapters of the Alzheimer's Association in your state can be very helpful in identifying trainers, resource material, and workshop opportunities. These chapters can be identified through the web site for the National Alzheimer's Association at www.alz.org.

Supervision

Supervision is the greatest precaution one can take against unsafe wandering. Assumptions that can be made when dealing with a cognitively-intact population of elders have little bearing when managing a cognitively impaired population. Staff really do need to feel that they need "eyes in the back of their heads" when they have responsibility for cognitively impaired elders. When staff are called away or need to answer a page, make sure that the transfer of responsibility for supervision is explicit. "I was watching Mrs. Jones water plants in the garden, could you take over until I return?" In addition, make sure that supervisory tasks are clearly understood when shifts change. Managing wandering behavior is a good example of where paying attention to details is extremely important. "I told Mrs. Jones to sit on the bench until I returned," would not be an adequate response to leaving a cognitively impaired elder unsupervised.

One would expect it reasonable that programs and services that have a direct mission to serve elders would be interested in heeding our concerns regarding dementia and wandering. Even if those settings were made safer than they are today in terms of trained staff and modifications to the physical environment, it would not be enough. Community residing elders with dementia do not spend their time in one place—their general routine may move them from home to day settings, but that routine is often interrupted by addressing acute health care concerns.

Acute Care Providers

Step back and think about all of the health care providers we encounter when we face a health concern—the general practice physician, the medical specialists, the nurses, the dentist, the dental specialists, the technicians, the receptionists. Do we know the professionals who treat us or are they new to us? How familiar are they with our medical conditions and with us as individuals? What is handled as an inpatient? What is treated on an outpatient basis? What support staff exist? Are they prepared to meet the needs of a patient who might wander away from a reception area, emergency room, or hospital bed? Do they know about community-based programs and services that have staff members who are trained in dementia care in order to make appropriate referrals?

Therapeutic design

Day, Carreon, and Stump (2000) reviewed the empirical literature on therapeutic design of environments for people with dementia. In commenting on safety, they noted that residents' attempts to leave facilities present a major concern for staff and family members. "Design solutions that prevent unwanted exiting often do so by exploiting residents' cognitive deficits" (p. 408). Is it really "exploiting" or is it meeting and understanding the individual's own reality?

For example, a full-length mirror placed in front of an exit door reduced residents' exit attempts by half in a study by Mayer and Darby (1991, in Day, et al., 2000). Another example is provided by Hussian and Brown (1987, in Day, et al., 2000) who observed a design strategy that capitalized on problems with depth perception—interpreting two-dimensional floor patterns as three-dimensional barriers. In their study, most exit attempts for some residents were eliminated. In a later study by Dickinson, McLain-Kark, and Marshall-Baker (1995, in Day, et al., 2000) a decrease in exit attempts from special care units was observed when closed, matching mini-blinds that restricted light and views through exit doors were installed. Other design strategies that depended on optical illusions to reduce unwanted exiting were camouflaging doorknobs, panic bars, and windows in exit doors—all seemed to help in eliminating exit attempts for most residents (Dickinson, et al., 1995, in Day, et al., 2000; Namazi, Rosner, & Calkins, 1989, in Day, et al., 2000).

Day and colleagues (2000) also reported on the success of studies by Hussian (1982–83, in Day, et al., 2000) in reducing exit attempts by conditioning residents to respond to attention-getting signage. Doors and stairways that had large colorful signs were avoided. Day and colleagues (2000) further noted that "accommodating residents' exit attempts, rather than discouraging them, also generated positive outcomes" (p. 409). Unlocking doors to secure outside areas helped to reduce agitation—reduced agitation was tied to increased autonomy as well as to increased outdoor usage (Namazi & Johnson, 1992, in Day, et al., 2000). The message here is that opportunities should be created to increase the autonomy of individuals with dementia by maximizing the safety of the area on the other side of the exit—the outdoor space.

Opportunity for easy surveillance was also noted in the review by Day, et al. (2000) as essential in maintaining safe environments (Morgan & Stewart, 1999, in Day, et al., 2000). Although an interesting observation noted by Lawton, Fulcomer, and Kleban (1984, in Day, et al., 2000) was that facilities where surveillance was too easily done may have minimized direct staff contact with residents. Our response to that observation is that it likely depends on the quality of the interactions—were they negative interactions (staff running after potential wanderers) or positive interactions (sharing in a meaningful activity)?

Restraint use

At the heart of the risk and autonomy debate is the issue of restraints. Shedd, Kobokovich, and Slattery (1995) observed in a study of 843 patients that confused patients (about 10% of the sample) were more likely to have either chemical or physical restraints than to have a sitter (a paid staff member or a family member who monitored the patient directly). In addition, confused patients were more likely to be discharged to an institution whereas nonconfused patients were discharged to their home or home with a visiting nurse referral. This is consistent with reports by Tangalos and others who state that for every day in a hospital, 3 to 5 days of rehabilitation are necessary to return to prehospitalization routine (Tangalos, 1999).

Hall (1999) offers several suggestions for avoiding restraints with confused adults who are hospitalized.

- Limit number of visitors and staff in the room at the same time
- No TV—human stimulus only
- Night-lights in bedroom and bathroom
- Scrupulous pain management
- Place bed in low position
- If patient is (or has been) married, line spouse's side of bed with pillows
- Rest periods alternating with activity throughout the day
- Consistent staff and routine
- Keep glasses, hearing aid, and dentures on
- Have purse (empty) in bed with patient
- Provide opportunities for chair rest during the day
- Provide meaningful activities
- Physical therapy to keep patient walking throughout the hospitalization
- Walk with the patient. If the patient *walked in*, make every effort to let them walk throughout the hospitalization and *walk out* at discharge
- Let family members stay with the patient around the clock

Diagnostic procedures

Routine activities in the hospital are not typically dementia-friendly. Day, Musallam, and Wells (1999) examined behaviors of hospitalized patients with probable Alzheimer's disease undergoing invasive diagnostic procedures. They concluded that routine assessment of the patients' usual behaviors, caregivers' knowledge of the stage of the disease, and awareness of the potential impact that diagnostics may have on cognitively impaired patients could help medical staff decide what interventions would most likely lead to successful outcomes. Of interest, is that wandering was noted in the records of 17% of the patients in their study (n = 30). Moreover, "restlessness" and "increased confusion" (both behaviors associated with the likelihood to wander) were recorded in 80% and 73% of the patients' charts respectively. Some hospitals have begun to address the special needs of individuals with dementia who require hospitalization.

Cabrini Medical Center in Manhattan opened their subunit, "Windows to the Heart" in April, 2000. This unit promotes an individualistic manner of care to each patient and his/her caregivers. The unit's staff is composed of nursing, social services, case management, chaplaincy, environmental services, homecare, and dietary. Each staff member completes 8 months of specialized training in dementia care and teamwork. The staff arranges with families to schedule X-rays and other tests and procedures at a time when family members can be present. Greater attention is also paid to delivering and clearing meal trays, and assisting with meals. The unit has open visiting hours and families (or professional caregivers) can spend time in a special lounge area that has a shower and kitchenette for their use (Alzheimer's Association, *New York City Chapter Newsletter*, 2000).

However, most hospitals are far behind the vision of Cabrini. An exploratory study of 32 hospitals in Massachusetts (Silverstein, et al., 2000) provided some insight into the hospital experience for people with dementia in that state. That study specifically asked the question, "How dementia-friendly are acute care hospitals?" The in-person interviews with directors of patient care were designed to gather data on current practices and planned changes related to dementia care as well as their perceptions about the major challenges hospitals faced in providing care to patients with dementia. While none of those surveyed was able to give specific statistics on the prevalence of patients with dementia admitted to their hospitals, 45% indicated that they had observed an increase in the numbers of patients with dementia who were admitted within the past 5 years. Only 3% had felt that the number of dementia patients had decreased. When asked if staff had received specialized training in dementia care, 5 hospitals (15%) reported that no specific training was offered in dementia care. The majority of the hospitals noted that they conducted training as part of their in-service or orientation programs. Only 9% of those surveyed were aware of the "Safe Return" program, the wanderers' alert program sponsored by the national Alzheimer's Association. None of the hospitals reported having a specific policy or protocol in place to refer to when a patient wandered away. Several respondents noted adaptations in practice or in the environment that they had made. Almost all, 97%, reported that they "select a room in a quieter area of the nursing unit where the patient has to pass by the nursing station before reaching an exit." Over half (58%) positioned the bed to "minimize visible cues of exits." Other adaptations noted by interviewees in this study were the use of alarms or buzzers, regular patient checks or "sweeps," alarm strips placed on bed and chairs, and wanderers' gowns (separate color than usual hospital gowns). Hall (1999) has suggested using a red vest as an "elopement identifier."

Dementia-friendly hospitals

The North Carolina Department of Health and Human Services Division on Aging (March, 2000) produced a guidebook on acute hospitalization and Alzheimer's disease. Several tips for hospital staff are offered in the guidebook and are useful in terms of minimizing the occurrence of unsafe wandering behavior in hospital settings and harmful consequences:

- Do not leave the patient alone in the emergency room or admissions lobby. A family member, trusted caregiver, or friend should be present at all times.
- Avoid numerous room changes. Change increases confusion and anxiety.
- Avoid patient rooms located in high-noise and high-traffic areas.
- Place the patient in a room that allows for easy and careful observation.
- Place patient in a room that is away from the stairs or elevator and not in eyesight.
- Place the patient in a room where he or she has to pass the nursing station in order to reach an exit.
- Have a photo of the patient on file.
- Assess the patient for pain and treat if needed.
- Ask the family member where and when the patient usually wanders. Find out what strategies have worked at home (or setting where patient was at prior to hospitalization).
- Keep the patients' suitcase, street shoes, and street clothes out of sight.
- Plan walks with the patient.
- Use distractions such as a snack or music.
- Take time to talk with the patient.
- Offer a simple, meaningful activity.

What we ask of acute health care providers is to expand their focus beyond the acute care need that presents itself. Dementia can clearly interfere with treatment if it is not considered in the care plan. The acute care environment can heed lessons learned in long-term care settings about caring for individuals who are cognitively impaired. Chapter 6 described what the current response to wandering behavior has been in long-term care settings and chapter 9 gleans recommendations from that current knowledge of best practice.

CHAPTER 10

The Lifesaving Role of "First Responders:" Recommendations for Police, EMS, Fire, and Search & Rescue Personnel

Some of the material in this chapter is adapted from *Law Enforcement, Alzheimer's Disease & the Lost Elder* (Flaherty & Scheft, 1995). We have also included here some practical materials produced by Robert J. Koester of the Virginia Department of Emergency Services, and the Virginia Search and Rescue Council, which were made available for use in this book by the author. Though some items may repeat, they are worth repeating. The bulleted items and checklist, in particular, are intended as a quick reference for law enforcement agencies and other first responders in cases involving a subject with Alzheimer's disease or a related memory impairment. These cases require an aggressive law enforcement response. Searches for people with Alzheimer's or other dementing illnesses are high-urgency.

POLICE AND EMS

As documented in chapter 5, there is a significant chance that as first responders, police officers will receive reports of older people who are missing from their homes in the community or from facilities such as nursing homes, rest homes, assisted living residences, or adult day centers. Most officers and many emergency medical personnel will, at some point, come in contact with an elderly person out on the street, lost and confused. Officers may also become involved in cases of neglect or abuse of an elder. In all of these situations involving the elderly, they should consider the possibility of Alzheimer's disease or a related dementia.

Anticipate Police Involvement

It is also worth repeating that Alzheimer's disease and related dementing illnesses primarily affect the elderly. One major study estimates that 10% of all people over age 65 suffer from a dementing illness. Prevalence among for those over age 85 (among the fastest growing populations in America) is estimated to be a staggering 47%. A small percentage (from 1–10%) of people with Alzheimer's are younger, typically in their 40s, 50s, or early 60s.

An estimated 70% of people with dementia live in the community, with the remainder in elder care facilities. The Congressional Office of Technology Assessment (1990) estimates that, at the very least, 20% of those people with a dementing illness who live in the community are living alone. This is especially alarming, because a national survey conducted by the Alzheimer's Association (1990) indicated that less than 2% of those who live in the community, or their caregivers, receive any support services (e.g., meals-on-wheels, adult day care, or home health aid).

Keep in mind also that the typical caregiver at home is a woman in her 70s who has at least two chronic health problems. Being aware of these circumstances can help police officers understand how people with Alzheimer's wander from their homes and become lost. It may be because there is no one at home to help or supervise them. Often, it is because their spouses, physically frail themselves, are exhausted by the around-the-clock care and supervision all people with Alzheimer's eventually require.

It is important also to note that most lost Alzheimer patients will be on foot (almost 90% in the 1996 Silverstein & Salmons study, and 84% in the 2001 Rowe & Glover study).

Recognition: IDs

There are no field tests to determine if someone has Alzheimer's disease or a related dementing illness, so police officers must look for clues. The clearest and most immediate way to know if someone you have found wandering has Alzheimer's is to look for an ID bracelet with the words "memory impaired" on the back, or for a wallet card with the same message. This bracelet identifies the person with dementia as being registered in the national Safe Return program. The toll-free number 1-800-572-1122 is on the back of the bracelet.

Safe Return Program

As detailed in chapter 5, families should be advised to register patients in the Safe Return program, the Alzheimer's Association's wanderers alert program, which operates with the support of the U.S. Justice Department. For a onetime fee (currently $40), the patient's key information is placed in a central registry. Safe Return operates around the clock, 365 days a year.

When a patient wanders away from home or an institution and the 800 number is called, a representative from the Alzheimer's Association can begin working with the missing person's caregiver, police, and others to gather and fax critical information. Follow-up counseling and service referrals are also offered through the Safe Return program to address the situation which led the elder to wander in the first place.

On encountering a confused elder, keep in mind that few people with Alzheimer's actually wear an ID bracelet or necklace. If there is no explicit ID, check for other forms of identification such as a driver's license or wallet cards. If the person does not have a paper ID, check for personalized ID labels on inner and outer clothing.

Recognition: Behavior and mental status

In addition to checking for identification, pay attention to how the person looks, behaves, and interacts with you. As a first responder, keep in mind that people with Alzheimer's can be sick or injured but unable to communicate that information effectively. Keep your interview and assessment simple, be calm, and use a reassuring tone of voice—remember, people with Alzheimer's take their action cues from your words and your behavior.

Physical Clues

Consider the following clues in determining whether you are dealing with someone who may have Alzheimer's disease or a related illness:

- Blank facial expression
- Inappropriately dressed for the weather
- An unsteady gait

Note, however, that people with Alzheimer's may experience visual-spatial problems early in the disease process, and this can sometimes make them appear intoxicated. Also, people with Alzheimer's typically are in their 70s and 80s, and should not be confused with street people.

Psychological Clues

Alzheimer's damages short-term memory, in particular. Someone with the disease may experience any or all of the following problems:

- Have an unusually difficult time understanding your questions
- Have trouble finding the right words to describe things
- Repeat certain words or phrases
- Ask the same question over and again
- Be disoriented as to time and location
- Be confused about their own and others' identities
- Be unable to communicate at all
- Be delusional
- And, if very frightened, possibly be combative

Situational Clues

An elderly person reported or discovered in one of the following situations may be suffering from Alzheimer's:

Missing or found wandering—Wandering is the most life-threatening behavior associated with Alzheimer's disease. It is also one of the most common situations you will encounter or respond to among people with Alzheimer's and other dementias. Wandering can be caused by restlessness due to boredom, lack of exercise, confusion about time or a change in the physical environment, agitation caused by overstimulation (from crowds, noise, or an argument with a caregiver, for example), or fear caused by a delusion or hallucination. Studies estimate that 60 to 70% of Alzheimer patients will wander from their residences at some point in their illness.

It is our opinion that all people with Alzheimer's disease who can walk are at risk of wandering, and thus becoming missing persons. Most suffer from other serious medical problems in addition to their Alzheimer's disease and are on essential medications which they will likely not take with them when they wander away from home or a facility and become lost. All, if not found quickly, are at risk of death. Mortality rates have been estimated to be as high as 46% after 24 hours (Koester & Stooksburg, 1995). Their health problems and diminished mental capacity dramatically increase the risk of death or serious injury, especially after the first 24 hours.

Following are some less common situations in which police may encounter people with Alzheimer's disease:

- **False reports**—A person with Alzheimer's may report an "intruder" in the house, who turns out to be a wife or husband. Patients may also report thefts that did not occur, especially given that those with Alzheimer's can experience heightened suspiciousness.
- **Victimization**—A person with Alzheimer's is easy prey for con artists. These patients may also come to your attention when you get involved in legal actions like evictions and repossessions because they have forgotten, or just are not able, to pay bills.
- **Shoplifting**—Sometimes people with Alzheimer's simply forget that they have picked something up, that it is necessary to pay for the item, or even that they are in a store. Of course, not all elderly shoplifters have Alzheimer's, but police should consider that possibility, particularly if the elder appears disoriented.
- **Indecent exposure**—People with Alzheimer's often fidget with zippers and buttons, which can be misinterpreted. Many have also lost impulse control, so if it feels too hot, they may just take their clothes off. If they feel the need to go to the bathroom, they may just do it without realizing they are not in the bathroom.

Interaction With Someone Who May Have Alzheimer's

Behavior management

In virtually any interaction where the memory-impaired person does not require medical attention at a hospital, the object is to return the person safely to his or her caregiver. Be advised that homeless shelters are not designed or staffed to care for someone with Alzheimer's disease.

When interacting with someone you suspect has a dementing illness such as Alzheimer's disease, it will help to know something about the theory of *behavior management* in Alzheimer's care. Behavior management is often just common sense. Alzheimer's disease can prevent the brain from correctly processing what a cognitively well person accepts as reality. In their confusion, people with Alzheimer's look to you—your body language, your tone of voice—for cues as to what they should do.

For example: You find an elderly, confused man sitting on the sidewalk, and he simply won't get up. Try sitting down next to him. Calmly introduce yourself, agree with whatever he says, and then slowly get up. He will likely also get up. As you move toward your cruiser, he will now be more likely to follow you, and to follow your cues for him to get in. He may refuse to get out of the cruiser when you arrive at his home (or the police station or hospital). His reasons may not make sense. Correcting him will only cause him to become more confused. Instead, tell him that everything is okay, that there's food, and family, inside. And if he asks for his mother, who is probably long dead, tell him she'll be right along. Be respectful, be reassuring, but don't be afraid to gently humor him by momentarily entering his reality. This approach is based on what we know about the role of emotion in the brain. The ability to feel and express emotion is a brain function that lasts until the end of our days. The approach we suggest helps create positive emotions in someone with Alzheimer's disease. It works, and because of the nature of this disease, there is nothing disrespectful in such an approach.

"Catastrophic" reactions

To facilitate a safe return, you must ease the situation and avoid causing the person with Alzheimer's to have a "catastrophic reaction," best described as a sort of super anxiety attack. What most people would consider mildly stressful, like being stopped and questioned by a police officer, can be extremely upsetting to someone with Alzheimer's. The individual is most likely to break down sobbing and crying, but may also become frightened, try to get away, or become angry, very agitated and, in extreme cases, even aggressive. These are more accurately referred to as "reactive" behaviors to what the person with dementia perceives (or rather, misperceives) as a threatening or stressful environment.

Avoid restraints

Understandably, the use of handcuffs and other restraints is likely to cause a catastrophic reaction. You should take advantage of any leeway you can offer the patient to avoid handcuffs. In unusual cases, however, an Alzheimer's patient who is extremely frightened or upset may threaten his own or others' safety. In this situation, restraint may be the best alternative for maintaining order. But bear in mind that, as a rule, these are frail people in their 70s and

80s. When it is absolutely necessary to restrain a memory-impaired elder, practice techniques for preventing injury. Even in cases of apparent domestic abuse, where statutes mandate certain standard responses, officers are still generally allowed some discretion as to whether or not to arrest a seriously memory-impaired elder.

Keep the climate cool

If you keep your voice calm and speak in a reassuring manner, you may help the memory-impaired person, and others involved, to do the same. This is why it is also important to use nonthreatening hand gestures. It is important to be firm, but nonaggressive. Again, reassurance works better than most current medications in treating this disease. This posture will help you draw the most helpful response from someone with Alzheimer's.

Keep communication simple

If possible, you should speak to the individual one on one, away from crowds and noise. Overloading the person with too much information in the middle of too much commotion may lead to a catastrophic reaction. Keep the following important considerations in mind:

- **Approach from the front and introduce yourself**—Do your best not to surprise the person when you approach him. Be sure he sees you. Tell him who you are and why you are there. You may have to explain several times because the person may not remember, from moment to moment, what you think should be obvious.
- **Speak slowly and calmly**—In order to hold the person's attention, look directly into his eyes as you speak.
- **Ask only one question and give only one direction at a time**—Try to ask simple questions. Do not ask questions which require a lot of thought and memory. Think of the brain in these cases as a sort of "overloaded switchboard" with incoming calls not always plugged into the right circuit. And remember, the person's answers may not reflect what he really means to say. As one patient put it, "It's as if I hear things and they get into the wrong slots, which make no sense to me at all."
- **Keep your instructions positive**—For example, say, "Please sit here in the car. Everything will be okay." Don't say things like, "Sit there and be quiet until I come back and don't try to get out of the car."

Try to avoid instructions requiring the subject to do, or think about, more than one simple thing at a time.

- **If necessary, repeat instructions**—If the person does not respond to what you say, wait a few moments and then repeat what you said earlier. The person may not remember what certain words mean, so it helps to reinforce your earlier statement.
- **Do not assume the person is hearing impaired**—Some 50% of people with Alzheimer's are indeed hearing-impaired. But shouting will probably not help them understand the meaning of your words. It may even frighten or agitate them, because they are taking their cues from your body language and tone of voice, and shouting could make you appear angry.

Police and the Alzheimer's Network

Essential orientation

What cannot be emphasized enough—even at the risk of seeming repetitious—is that a missing person with Alzheimer's disease represents an emergency situation. Police cannot invoke any waiting period before taking action. Such a delay might be appropriate in the case of a missing young adult who is apparently competent to make his or her own decisions and has the ability to function in the community. But, sadly, the ability of people with Alzheimer's simply to find their way from one point to another and back again is impaired very early in the disease process. Additionally, they are at high risk of dehydration and hypothermia. Their judgment is impaired, their health may be seriously impaired, and they are also at risk of a catastrophic reaction at any time when lost, especially as darkness approaches. And if safety reasons were not enough, consider the psychological terror of being lost and unable to think through what to do about it. Take these cases seriously.

Notification: How police learn about wanderers

You will encounter or learn about Alzheimer's wanderers in three different ways:

The Street Encounter

As discussed previously, you will at some time encounter an Alzheimer's patient during patrol or while answering a call thought to involve a different kind of issue—a man reported walking aimlessly at night on the shoulder of a busy road, for example, or a strange woman reported sitting in the lobby of a building, or a routine auto accident—but you soon discover that the man, the woman, or the driver is elderly and very confused. In these instances you try to identify the elders and return them safely to their caregivers.

Where identification is a problem, it is advisable to contact the Alzheimer's Association Safe Return operator (1-800-572-1122), who will check for a possible match in the Safe Return registry and can advise experienced, area on-call personnel in the program to alert the elder service network in surrounding communities.

Even in cases where the situation is more easily resolved, it is also highly advisable to alert Safe Return, which keeps valuable records of such wandering episodes, so that professional staff at the local chapter can assess the situation which resulted in the person's wandering and offer counseling to the patient and his family. The Alzheimer's Association chapter can also encourage the development of a service plan to cover any gaps in care or supervision of the patient. Be advised that wandering and becoming lost is often a repeated behavior.

Caregiver Notifies the Police

A second scenario occurs when a caregiver calls police to request assistance in finding a missing elder who may be memory-impaired.

Collect information—When you receive a call from a caregiver about a missing Alzheimer's patient, be sure to obtain the following information:

- Caller's name, phone and address
- Length of time missing
- Whether the missing person is registered with Safe Return and wearing the program bracelet
- Is person carrying any ID, money, credit or ATM cards
- Where last seen. (And whether person has disappeared before. If so, where found)
- Physical appearance, clothing
- Medical condition, medications
- Whether on foot or driving (If driving, make, model, year, color, and plate number)
- Whether the person can communicate (Does person know own name, address, speak English)
- Did the person appear to be agitated before disappearance

- Was the immediate area searched. (If not, request that caller have someone do so immediately, or have caller do so. If at all possible, however, someone at the caller's residence should try to remain by the phone.)

Call Safe Return Program—You should then contact the operator at the Safe Return program at the toll-free number, 1-800-572-1122, to communicate the information you collected. You should also anticipate the distribution of key information, since the Safe Return operator will fax a report to the local police and hospital. In some areas of the country, there are more extensive fax communication networks which local Safe Return staff can access immediately. Where available, this network is capable of broadcasting hundreds of faxes at once. In these cases, fax alerts containing pertinent information can go to all police departments in a given area, including transit police (an important notification since some missing elders will be capable of accessing public transportation), and state police (an important notification since some missing elders who are driving may enter interstate highways); hospital emergency rooms; EMS and ambulance services; local shelters; and Medical Examiners' offices.

Cooperate with the Local Chapter of the Alzheimer's Association—The Association's national Safe Return operator will call or fax a report to the local Association chapter during normal office hours and can notify local on-call personnel after hours in some areas to assist the police in coordinating efforts to find the missing patient. You may want to speak directly with staff at the local chapter to seek their assistance and expertise, which you can do through the national Safe Return operator. (In nonemergencies during regular business hours, you can call the local chapter number directly. To locate your local chaper, check: www.alz.org.)

Caregiver Notifies the National Alzheimer Safe Return Program

A third situation arises when a caregiver calls Safe Return before calling police. The procedure is similar to that outlined above. The Safe Return operator, having received the caregiver's call, will obtain the requisite information, advise the caller to notify the local police immediately, and will then fax a report to the local police. The Safe Return operator can also provide any additional information which may be helpful, particularly if the missing person is registered in the program. Note that the program will respond whether or not the missing memory-impaired elder is registered in Safe Return.

The Association's local staff will contact the reporting caregiver (typically a family member) to verify that the patient is still lost, and to further discuss the circumstances. The local staff may also contact local police to discuss any additional appropriate response to the situation, including use of the more extensive fax alert network where available.

Operations: The Police Search and Related Responsibilities

The police have two major responsibilities when confronted with a missing person report concerning someone who may have Alzheimer's disease. They must first handle communications and, second, conduct an appropriate search.

Communications

Certain kinds of communications are critical. Police must:

- Place the report on the NCIC (the U.S. Justice Department's National Crime Information Center) computer network. Be sure to check NCIC to see if the information has been logged appropriately. If not, make sure that this is done.
- Issue radio report to surrounding communities. Do not assume that a fax transmittal is a substitute for radio contact. Most police patrol officers use the radio as their immediate source of information and, especially in cases of lost Alzheimer's patients, time is of the essence.
- Ask neighboring police departments to include a report in all shift briefings.
- Notify change of shifts at your own department. Take responsibility for ensuring that future shifts are notified about the missing Alzheimer's patient. Failure to inform future shifts can affect the continuity of the search process.
- Inform media outlets. Media outlets—especially TV and radio news stations—should be notified immediately if any of the following conditions apply:

    1. The missing person has a life-threatening health problem.
    2. The weather is extremely cold or hot.
    3. Darkness begins to fall.
    4. The report comes in at night, the person has been missing for more than 2 hours, and an effort has already been made to find him.

- When appropriate, access state emergency management resources. These state agencies have ground and air search and rescue capabilities which can be utilized for missing elders. This service may be especially useful in rural and some suburban areas. The local police department must request these services, generally after having used available local resources in the search effort. (See more on search and rescue, below.)
- Notify local postal officials. Postal officials can alert mail carriers, who provide an excellent network of eyes and ears in the community where the missing person may still be wandering, lost and confused.

The search

Officers should search the immediate and surrounding areas first—and double check the person's residence. If possible, return every few hours to the immediate area where the person was last seen. When on foot, most missing persons with Alzheimer's disease are located within a fairly short distance—usually no more than a mile from where they disappeared. Many are found in neighbors' yards and on streets close to home.

Be sure to check those places most familiar to the person, such as a former neighborhood or past place of employment, a relative's home, a regularly attended place of worship, a frequented shopping place, a favorite restaurant.

In rural areas, the person is often found a short distance from a road or open field, near a creek or drainage ditch, or tangled in underbrush. It is important to know that missing persons with Alzheimer's disease are not likely to respond to shouts and will not cry out for help.

Below is some additional helpful guidance excerpted (with permission) from Koester (Alzheimer's and Related Disorders Missing Person Checklist for Police Version 1.5, March 3, 2001, produced with the support and collabo ration of The Virginia Center of Aging Grant 97-02):

Initial Officer/Deputy Actions

- ❒ Collect initial report.
- ❒ Determine degree of physical search warranted.

If Physical Search Is Warranted

- ❒ Identify and secure the Point Last Seen (PLS) or Last Known Position (LKP) as a crime scene.
    - ❒ Place barrier tape.

- ❐ Secure scent article.
- ❐ Secure tracks.
- ❐ Remove or stop idling engines.

- ❐ Contact shift supervisor and/or SAR coordinator, request additional resources.
- ❐ Search residence and grounds if applicable, regardless of previous efforts.
- ❐ Patrol immediate area.

Additionally, there are useful models of police response to reports of missing persons with Alzheimer's disease. The Boston Police, for example, in cooperation with the Boston Commission on Affairs of the Elderly and the Alzheimer's Association's Massachusetts Chapter, have instituted a thorough procedure to deal with all missing elderly residents and Alzheimer's patients. These procedures (outlined in Special Order #92-2) apply to Boston residents who: 1) are suspected of suffering from Alzheimer's disease or other memory impairment; 2) are of poor mental health; or 3) are 60 years of age or older.

Notification

When a missing person report is received, the responding officer must notify the Boston Commission on Affairs of the Elderly through the Mayor's 24-hour Hotline. (Although not formally mentioned in the rule, officers can access the Safe Return program in the manner discussed above.)

Reporting and searching

In all cases, a complete intake is done, and appropriate reports filed, in order to activate both a Police Department response and the NCIC network. The appropriate Area Commander, in conjunction with a Senior Response Unit Officer (one such officer is assigned to each area command), then coordinates a search for the missing individual.

Follow-up

What is perhaps most impressive about the Boston model is its emphasis on effective follow-up with the individual who reported the missing person. The Special Order, which resulted from the highly publicized deaths of two Alzheimer's wanderers in Boston in 1991, mandates that the Area Commander must ensure:

1) That an officer contacts or visits the individual who made the initial report at least once each day for 5 days after a report is received, and ascertain whether the missing elder has returned or been recovered; and 2) that after the initial 5-day period, an officer visits the informant at least once a week until the elder has been located. The officer's name and the date and time of each contact must be recorded on the missing person report.

POLICE, FIRE, AND SEARCH & RESCUE PERSONNEL

> Handled chiefly on a local level, (search and rescue) procedures for locating wandering elderly people with dementia are a chink in the armor of the system. We don't do this well.
>
> —Curt Rudge, Chief of Ranger Services
> Massachusetts Department of Emergency Management
> From *The Boston Globe* (December 25, 1999)

In the above quote, Rudge offers expert testimony about the frustration of search and rescue professionals who are consulted or called out to search for Alzheimer's wanderers too late to put their skills at saving lives to work. In fact, in late 1996, Rudge was involved in two cases in which missing Alzheimer's patients died. Neither missing person was registered in Safe Return, and the program did not learn about either case for several days. By that time, more than 100 searchers had already been involved in each of the cases. Yet it was not until Rudge arrived with another state Park Ranger and their two air-scent dogs (at the encouragement of the Safe Return program in Massachusetts and by invitation of local police) that either body was found. Both missing persons are assumed to have died within 24 hours of having been reported missing. Both were found roughly within half a mile of the point where they were positively last seen. Both were found in dense bush or briars.

In addition to the earlier guidance provided for law enforcement personnel to aid in their response to reports of missing elders who may be suffering from memory impairments, this chapter also contains useful recommendations for search and rescue personnel. These recommendations are based principally on a study of the Virginia Department of Emergency Services database and on data collected under search conditions (Koester & Stooksbury, 1995), which resulted in several critical observations of special use for search planners. The thumbnail sketch of the two cases cited above, and our experience in other cases, is very consistent with the Koester and Stooksbury search and rescue (SAR) research review adapted further on in this chapter.

Koester was the first to report a statistical search profile of the Alzheimer's disease patient. He also showed that healthy elderly and Alzheimer's patients must be treated as having two separate profiles. And in a finding consistent with our experience, he reports that:

> On some searches the caregiver emphatically stated the lost subject "does not have Alzheimer's disease." Yet instead, the lost subject suffered from vascular dementia or Parkinson's dementia. Both of which may be equally severe. At this time, it appears the nature of wandering, from a search perspective, is the same for all the Alzheimer's and related diseases. (From Koester at www.dbs-sar.com)

Koester's findings, summarized below, are thoroughly supported by our own research and case experience, portions of which are represented in these important behavioral observations. One such observation cited by Koester was reported rather poignantly by a lost Alzheimer's patient: "I go until I get stuck." The sticking point, in our experience, can refer either to a physical barrier such as a fence or other impasse, or to a perceived barrier, such as darkness. The very perception of a barrier can trigger a "catastrophic reaction," the super anxiety attack referenced earlier, which further diminishes the person's ability to negotiate his or her way to a safe place. Further, Koester has found that lost persons with Alzheimer's disease appear to lack the ability to turn around, or reverse their direction, a phenomenon consistent with the finding by Duffy, Tetewsky & O'Brien (2000) that people with Alzheimer's have difficulty "remapping" their route back to the starting point.

The Lost Alzheimer's Subject: SAR Research Review

- Subjects with Alzheimer's disease leave few physical clues.
- Subjects often have a previous history of wandering (72%).
- Subjects may attempt travel to a former residence or to a favorite place.
- Mobility is commonly limited by coexisting medical problems.
- Often the last sighting is on a roadway.
- 67% crossed or departed from roads.
- The median distance traveled was 0.5 miles (in contrast to 2.5 miles for healthy elderly persons), as measured in a straight line.
- The 90% probability zone (for distance traveled) was 0 to 1.1 miles, and the 96% probability zone was 0 to 1.5 miles.

- Subjects were usually found a short distance from a road or open field (50% within 33 yards).
- 63% of subjects were found in creek or drainage areas and/or caught in briars or bushes.
- Subjects will not cry out for help or respond to shouts from searchers (only 1% did so).
- All subjects located within 24 hours of the time last seen were found alive (although cold weather can have a significant negative impact on this outcome).
- 46% of subjects did not survive after 24 hours from the time they were last seen alive. (Hill, 1991, supports this high fatality rate, reporting a mortality rate of 45% [10 of 22 subjects] among "walkaways.")
- Most subjects died as a result of hypothermia, dehydration, and/or drowning.

Searching for people with Alzheimer's disease who have wandered and become lost is one of the most critical services provided by law enforcement. A report to the Virginia House of Delegates prepared by the Virginia Department of Criminal Justice Services (2000) states that the department's survey of police chiefs and county sheriffs found that nearly 80% had been involved in searches for lost Alzheimer's patients. While 80% of these missing patients were found safe, 20% were found either injured or deceased. The critical factor cited in the report was the time it took to find the missing patient.

> Of all cases, over one-third of the patients not found within 24 hours were found deceased. Conversely, of those individuals found within 12 hours, none were found deceased or injured. Thus, it is critical that law enforcement be trained properly and respond immediately to situations involving Alzheimer's patients (p. 11).

One method of response suggested by search and rescue experts is called "reflex tasking." Reflex tasks can be described as the initial rapid deployment of resources into the most likely areas where the subject may have wandered (Koester, 1999). Based on what is known about the profile of the missing Alzheimer's subject, Koester suggests the following reflex tasks. Some are within the domain of law enforcement agencies, some more appropriate to trained search and rescue personnel. As with any checklist, some items may not always apply, additional steps may be required, or the order in which the tasks are performed may vary. And as with any profession, search and rescue has its own shorthand. Note a few abbreviations: Point Last Seen (PLS), the site the missing person was positively last seen by a reliable source; Point Last Known, the site where the missing person is assumed to have most recently been (e.g., if the missing person was driving a car which is later found unoccupied, the PLK would be the car); Initial Planning Point (IPP), the site where the search starts, which can be the PLS, PLK, or other site most practical for the search team.

Reflex Tasks

- ❒ Conduct a highly systematic search of residence/nursing home and grounds (required of law enforcement).
- ❒ Send patrols to areas where the subject has been previously located.
- ❒ As an investigative task, canvas neighborhood.
- ❒ Patrol along roads. Patrol should extend to the theoretical search area, especially in urban environments.
- ❒ Establish containment points.
- ❒ Use trackers (early) at the PLS.
- ❒ Use tracking dogs (early) at the IPP, along roadways, or at any area where clues are found.
- ❒ Deploy air-scent dog teams into drainages and streams, starting at sites nearest the IPP.
- ❒ Deploy hasty ground teams (early) into drainages and streams nearest the IPP.
- ❒ "Cut for sign" (i.e., look for where the subject may have left the road) along roadways.
- ❒ Have dog teams and ground sweep teams (in separate sectors) expand from the IPP. Ensure that teams search heavy briars/bushes.
- ❒ Have air-scent dog teams and ground sweep teams search 100 yards (initially) in from and parallel to roadways.
- ❒ Search nearby previous homesites and the region between homesites and the IPP.
- ❒ Repeat search of residence/nursing home grounds at least twice a day.
- ❒ Post flyers in appropriate locations.
- ❒ After initial tasks, the search should expand outward from the IPP.

Note that personal locator technology is sometimes effective in these searches. For more on this technology, see chapter 5.

AUTOMOBILES, ALZHEIMER'S AND THE POLICE

Alzheimer's disease affects reaction time and visual-spatial relationships. Because they may be driving—yet unaware of the severity of their disease—

people with Alzheimer's can easily become lost or even leave the scene of an accident after literally forgetting what happened. Studies of people in the early stage of the disease who were still driving indicate that over 40% had been in a car crash and 44% routinely got lost (for more on driving issues, see chapter 7). Police should let the Department of Motor Vehicles know their concerns in cases of confused or disoriented elders who are driving, and are also advised to contact the local Alzheimer's Association so that counselors can advise the drivers' families or other caregivers.

Silverstein and Murtha's (2001) study provides additional insight to law enforcement by drawing on the comments made by the officers who were interviewed about older drivers.

> The person thought that the light was green when, in fact, it was red. The driver hit two pedestrians in the crosswalk. (p. 12)

> Many motor vehicle accidents are caused by elderly drivers who consistently think that the brake is the gas petal. They get confused. I think a yearly test should be administered to drivers who are over the age of 70. (p. 17)

Yet, when respondents were then asked whether they considered the statement "Police officers are reluctant to issue tickets or warnings to older drivers" to be true or false, the general public and physicians were more likely to feel that police officers are not reluctant to ticket older drivers, while police officers, themselves, were more likely to agree that police officers are reluctant ($p < .001$). The following comment from a police officer seems to illustrate this reluctance:

> "Just last week I had a 94-year-old with an expired inspection sticker. He bragged at how old he was. I let him go."

Driving and aging is an issue that extends beyond dementia and driving. We emphasize the concern here because we have made several references throughout this book to wandering and driving. While colleagues may argue that individuals in the early stages of dementia can safely operate a vehicle, we should all keep two questions in mind:

- Can these drivers reach their destination and return home safely?
- How do we know when they have passed the threshold from "safe early stage driver" to "unsafe driver?"

When dementia is formally diagnosed, or it is suspected that the executive functioning associated with driving ability is compromised, we suggest that alternative forms of transportation be pursued.

Kulash (2000) noted that "greater cooperation and specific procedures between the medical community and licensing agents are required. A prototype referral system for medical, legal, and licensing practitioners should be developed and evaluated" (p. 32). A clear pathway for referral, assessment, and licensure does not currently exist in most states.

Several of the findings from the Silverstein and Murtha (2001) study provide additional support for some of the recommendations already put forward by the U.S. Department of Transportation and the National Highway Traffic Safety Administration, specifically to "encourage creative partnerships among elder advocates, governments, care providers, insurers, and others, and develop better rehabilitation and regulation of drivers" (Kulash, 2000, p. 9).

The New York State Office for the Aging published a handbook, *When You Are Concerned: A Guide for Families Concerned About the Safety of an Older Driver* (LePore, 2000). The handbook was funded by the New York State Governor's Traffic Safety Committee and by the Allstate Insurance Foundation and additionally supported by the New York State Department of Motor Vehicles, New York State Police, and the New York State Department of Health. All states should consider such a public awareness campaign. We would also encourage the development of companion handbooks, such as *When You Are Concerned: A Guide for Physicians* and *When You Are Concerned: A Guide for Law Enforcement.*

In addition, Silverstein and Murtha (2001) suggest that more education and training be provided for police officers to sensitize them to older drivers and to the complications that can arise because of failure to cite or ticket, which inadvertently sanctions unsafe driving. The implication here is that the driver will benefit from early detection of unsafe driving and referrals for appropriate intervention.

SUMMARY

Increasingly, police officers are dealing with people in the community who have Alzheimer's disease or another type of dementia. Effective intervention is a challenge for both the individual officer and for the department.

Officers must demonstrate compassion and good judgment when interacting with people who, through no fault of their own, may be extremely difficult to communicate with and to gather information from. Despite that frustration, they should remember to keep calm, to keep things in perspective and, just as important, to keep their sense of humor. People with Alzheimer's disease are members of our society who should be valued and respected. They have lost their memories, not their need for protection.

As neurologist A. R. Luria wrote to Oliver Sacks: "Man does not consist of memory alone. He has feeling, will, sensibility, moral being. It is here you may touch them, and see a profound change" (Sacks, 1985).

As with other issues affecting law enforcement and other first responders, a coordinated response is the most effective approach. Police are encouraged to use the Alzheimer's Association's national Safe Return network. The Association has developed expertise to help find missing memory-impaired elders and to assist in adjusting any caregiving conditions which may have precipitated an elder's disappearance. There is another benefit of utilizing the national Safe Return network. Once you or another source notifies the Safe Return 800 operator that the missing Alzheimer's patient is located, the program will verify the report and then authorize a fax alert to the previously notified agencies and outlets to inform them that the search is over. This saves countless hours of wasted effort and phone calls. The local Association chapter will also refer recovered patients and their families to other support and resources available in their communities.

Conclusions

We hope that the reader now shares our concerns about dementia and wandering. Dementia poses challenges to our assumptions about our daily lives. These challenges to occur for the individual, his or her family and friends, formal care providers, and the larger community.

The individual with early stage dementia will need help to recognize that his or her driving capacity has diminished and to plan for alternative forms of transportation. Registering in the Safe Return wanderer's alert program is also a proactive step that the individual in the early stages of dementia may take for him or herself as well. Wearing a Safe Return bracelet can provide some reassurance to the early-stage individual as well as to caregivers as the disease progresses.

Family members and friends are challenged because they know an individual's history of past behavior and want to assume that what happened before is a blueprint for what will happen next. We know that that is not the case with dementia. Family members are surprised by behaviors exhibited that were never characteristic of the individual before the disease. The message in this book is that caregivers should expect the unexpected. Knowing that "it is the disease" and not something the individual with dementia is intentionally doing may help family members and friends continue to offer support rather than avoid contact with the individual and his or her primary caregiver. Caregivers who recognize an individual's potential for wandering and getting lost will take precautions to minimize the likelihood of it occurring. That has implications for the caregiver in terms of modifying the home environment and changing the caregiver's own responsibilities and routine.

Formal care providers are challenged because caring for a cognitively impaired elder population requires specialized training that differs from providing care to an exclusively physically frail elder population. Experience and skills in working with elders in general do not necessarily transfer to working with elders who have dementia. The chapters in this book should help those who work in the elder service network to understand where there are differences in approaches to care and how they might seek training opportunities that address those approaches. In addition, adaptations may be needed in the physical environments in which services are delivered.

Increased community awareness of dementia and, specifically, of wandering as a high-risk behavior, will aid search and rescue efforts when a cognitively impaired elder does wander away and become lost. We do not want people to "look the other way" when they see an elder who is noticeably confused or dressed inappropriately for the weather conditions.

IMPLICATIONS FOR PRACTICE AND POLICY

Reaching out to Caregivers

Caregivers may employ a wait-and-see strategy and respond only in the event of a crisis rather than in time for prevention (Silverstein, Hyde, & Ohta, 1993). With these results in mind, the main recommendation to evolve from our exploration of this issue involves outreach to, and education of, formal and informal care providers. Such efforts should inform caregivers about what is known about wandering, in particular that it is a common symptom of the disease, that it can happen to anyone, and that it often occurs without warning. Risks associated with wandering should be publicized beyond the traditional networks. Educational materials and programs should also share the details about relatively easy and low-cost safeguards that can be taken—just in case.

Also related to education and outreach is the importance of finding individuals with dementia who live alone. These individuals are likely to have fewer precautions in place to minimize the likelihood of wandering away and becoming lost, and are less likely to have 24-hour supervision. Education efforts should help noncustodial caregivers understand that the person with Alzheimer's who is living alone may also be getting lost.

Increasing Awareness of Professionals and Paraprofessionals of the Risks Associated With Wandering Behavior

The level of professional and paraprofessional understanding concerning the risks of wandering behavior must also be increased. Home care, respite care, and adult day health care professionals would benefit from education about wandering and effective management techniques. Targeted outreach, education, and intervention programs for wandering and its prevention should be developed and implemented widely. Educational and training videos and materials on wandering and the Safe Return program are available through the Alzheimer's Association. In addition, individuals who are newly diagnosed should have Safe Return information and materials on wandering behavior available to them in their doctors' offices and diagnostic centers.

Developing Better Rehabilitation and Regulation of Drivers

We must expand opportunities for reassessment and road testing. To increase the likelihood that individuals take advantage of reassessment opportunities, we should explore policy options for reimbursement or reduced-rate offerings, if referred by physician. Kulash (2000) suggests a multiple-tier system of testing where the initial round of assessment serves as a screening tool and relies on simple, low-cost, easily administered tests. In-depth assessment would be conducted only if deficiencies were noted in the initial phase. This would avoid the cost and emotional burden of unnecessary testing. Kulash (2000) further notes that the AMA has recommended that "physicians should work with their state medical societies to create statutes that uphold the best interests of patients and community, and that safeguard physicians from liability when reporting in good faith" (p. 18). The following key recommendations of the American Medical Association (adapted from Kulash, 2000, p. 19) provide further guidance to the physicians' role:

1. Physicians should assess patients' physical or mental impairments that might adversely affect driving abilities. In making evaluations, physicians should consider the following factors:
   a. the physician must be able to identify and document physical or mental impairments that clearly relate to the ability to drive; and
   b. the driver must pose a clear risk to public safety.
2. Before reporting, there are a number of initial steps physicians should take.
   a. discuss with the patient and family the risks of driving;
   b. consider a restricted driving schedule;
   c. negotiate a workable plan that may render reporting unnecessary.
3. Physicians should use their best judgment when determining when

> to report impairments that could limit a patient's ability to drive safely. In situations where clear evidence of substantial driving impairment implies a strong threat to patient and public safety, and where the physician's advice to discontinue driving privileges is ignored, physicians have an ethical duty to notify their state's Department of Motor Vehicles.

Programs such as *DriveWise: A Driving Fitness Evaluation Program* offered through Beth Israel Deaconess Medical Center in Boston, offer a comprehensive evaluation of driving performance that includes a road test for individuals whose safety may be compromised due to impairments in motor, cognitive, perceptual, and sensory abilities (DriveWise, 2001). DriveWise provides a useful model for the assessment and remediation of driving problems. DriveWise is a collaborative effort involving an interdisciplinary team of health care professionals who work closely with one another in the evaluation and remediation of medically ill patients with driving problems. The team includes professionals from rehabilitation services, social work, and neuropsychology. Each professional provides expertise in his or her respective field that is critical in making a final set of recommendations to the patient, family, and physician regarding continued driving. While DriveWise was initially conceptualized to evaluate the older driver with dementia, the program has expanded its patient population to include other diagnostic groups of patients (e.g., traumatic brain injury, brain tumors, multiple sclerosis, and psychiatric problems). The program has a community based advisory board with representatives from the Alzheimer's Association, the Registry of Motor Vehicles, the state Department of Elder Affairs, AARP, and the state Department of Public Health. Team members from DriveWise are active in public speaking and education of other health care professionals to increase public awareness about this important issue (O'Connor & Kapust, 2001).

Balancing Concern Over Safety While Preserving Personal Autonomy

The person with dementia should be encouraged to participate in the decisions affecting his life for as long in the disease process as possible. Providing immediate and useful information to the person with early stage dementia and to his or her caregiver about the likelihood of wandering and the risks associated with that behavior can have an empowering impact on an individual's ability to plan for that likelihood. That sense of exercising some degree of self-determination is reflected in the following quotations from individuals participating in 2001 in an early stage patient support group in Massachusetts facilitated by Joanne Koenig-Coste:

> "I have learned to stop and ask for directions when I get lost on my daily walks. I even rang a stranger's bell. She told me I was one block from home. My husband bought a Nordic track. We keep it in the garage and sometimes I use that instead of walking outside and fearing becoming lost again."

> "Most of the time I forgot I had Alzheimer's in the earliest days until I realized one morning that I could not visually map out in my mind where I was supposed to go that day and it was a place I frequented. I had a hard time coming to grips with this loss of visual memory. It was this realization that made me talk to my family and get help. I have not worried about getting lost because, since that day, I do not leave the house by myself . . . never. To not be able to create a map in your mind is so scary."

> "When spaces look unfamiliar to me, I stop, take a deep breath, and try to gather my thoughts. As a physician, I have been trained not to panic and that has served me well when I feel lost. I have always had a remarkable sense of direction and on the few occasions when I felt lost driving I did this same exercise and fairly soon I spotted something familiar and found my way home. Then I decided that driving was just too risky and so I quit . . . sadly, but I quit."

While caregivers are very concerned about the safety of the person with Alzheimer's, they worry about preserving personal autonomy and independence for that person as well. This reality should be considered when suggesting management techniques and prevention strategies to caregivers. As demonstrated in the literature, recommendations for safety precautions are not likely to be implemented if they are not congruent with the values and beliefs of the caregiver (Roberto, 1994; Silverstein, Hyde, & Ohta, 1993). Moreover, the importance of the two competing ideas of safety and personal freedom should be recognized and incorporated into any intervention, education, or outreach effort. Any suggestions for effective prevention strategies should also include ones for managing the agitation, diverting the attention, and redirecting the focus of the person with Alzheimer's.

Designing and Implementing Helpful Interventions

Since there is currently no cure or lasting treatment for Alzheimer's and related dementias, interventions that help both the person with Alzheimers' and the caregiver in their daily lives are essential. Caregivers respond in a variety of ways to coping with the problem of wandering. For these reasons, intervention programs need to begin with an assessment that considers the lifestyle and needs of the caregiver, the preferred way of providing care, the needs of the person with Alzheimer's, and the needs of the household. Such an assessment would aid in the development of an appropriate and effective intervention that might also be more readily accepted by the caregiver. Finally, intervention efforts should also educate, instruct, and support caregivers in the implementation and use of precautions that can be used for the multiple safety problems they face, including wandering.

Many venues, including the Alzheimer's Association's Safe Return program and family support groups would seem to be appropriate and effective settings for the outreach, education, and intervention efforts recommended above. Current findings suggest that working with and through the police might be an effective conduit as well. In the Silverstein and Salmons (1996) study, more than half of the caregivers of those who had wandered had received some help from the police during the course of the wandering episode, although as previously noted only 27% had initiated that contact. In fact, the Safe Return program already works with police and other emergency personnel to train them to recognize and deal appropriately with people who have Alzheimer's disease. The wider aging network, from the Administration on Aging on a national level to the State Units on Aging, and down to the regional Area Agencies on Aging and local Councils on Aging can play a much stronger role in reaching individuals with dementia and their caregivers. Some states have Alzheimer's Advisory Councils or task forces that have greatly assisted with outreach on program and policy levels.

Promoting Caregivers' Use of Precautions for Minimizing the Effects of Unsafe Wandering

In the Silverstein and Salmons (1996) study, while almost all of the caregivers were using at least one precaution to address wandering behavior, only about 20% reported that they were using monitors or alarms. Of these, most were using homemade devices composed of chimes or bells. Only rarely did someone report using technological instruments or wandering-alert devices such as "sensor alarms." Several such devices have been proposed or are already on the market but are in limited use, including electronic tracking devices. Greater accessibility to technological devices may not only help to preserve the autonomy of people in the early stage of a dementing illness, but may also help to minimize the risk of injury due to wandering. Practical technology has the potential to provide them with a greater degree of freedom, while minimizing anxiety among their caregivers by making it possible for those who become lost to be found more quickly. At present, first responders, caregivers and patients alike are committing their physical and emotional resources to resolve a problem—wandering and getting lost—for which they know there is no single reliable solution. This is both draining and discouraging. An efficient and affordable technology that addresses the "no-solution syndrome" will likely win acceptance and save lives.

A final note—there is great promise emerging from the medical and scientific research communities that our future will hold a world without Alzheimer's disease. We look forward to that day. In the meantime, we are concerned about the four million or more individuals and their families in the United States, and the millions of others around the world, who are coping with dementing illnesses. We hope that through this book we have contributed to making their daily lives a little more manageable and a little less stressful.

References

Adler, G. (1997). Driving and dementia: Dilemmas and decisions. (Supplement: Alzheimer's Disease—A Multidisciplinary Challenge). *Geriatrics, 52*(9), p. S26 (4).

Albert, S. M. (1992). The nature of wandering in dementia: A Guttman scaling analysis of an empirical classification scheme. *International Journal of Geriatric Psychiatry, 7*, 783–787.

Algase, D. L. (1999). Wandering: A dementia-compromised behavior. *Journal of Gerontological Nursing, 25*(9), 10–17.

Algase, D. L. (1992). A century of progress: Today's strategies for responding to wandering behavior. *Journal of Gerontological Nursing, 18*(11), 28–34.

Algase, D. L. (1992b). Cognitive discriminants of wandering among nursing home residents. *Nursing Home Research, 41*(2), 78–81.

Allen, K. (1994). Dementia in acute units: Wandering. *Nursing Standard, 9*(8), 16–23.

Altus, D. E., Mathews, R. M., Xaverius, P. K., Engelman, K. K., & Nolan, B. A. (2000). Evaluating an electronic monitoring system for people who wander. *American Journal of Alzheimer's Disease and Related Disorders* (March/April), 121–125.

Alzheimer's Association. (2002). *General Statistics/Demographics.* Available at: http://www.alz.org.

Alzheimer's Association. (2002). *Safe return statistics.* Chicago, IL: Author.

Alzheimer's Association. (2001). *10 warning signs. Alzheimer's Disease and Related Disorders Association, Inc.* Available: http://www.alz.org.

Alzheimer's Association. (1997). *Community assessment workbook for dementia services.* Chicago, IL: Author.

Alzheimer's Association. (1992). The physical environment. In *Guidelines for dignity: Goals for specialized Alzheimer/dementia care in residential settings* (pp. 35–38). Chicago, IL: Author.

Alzheimer's Association. (1993). The challenges of wandering: Practical approaches precede research. *Research and Practice, 2*(3), 1–2.

Alzheimer's Association. (1991). Wandering: Keeping the person with Alzheimer's safe and secure. *National Newsletter, 11*(4), 3.

Alzheimer's Association. (2000). Dementia unit opens culture change in acute care. *New York City Chapter Newsletter, 17,* 1, 5.

Alzheimer's Association, Massachusetts Chapter. (2001). *Family Care Guide*. Cambridge, MA: Author.

Alzheimer's Association, Massachusetts Chapter. (1990). *Alzheimer's disease: The facts.* [Brochure]. Cambridge, MA: Author.

Alzheimer's Association, St. Louis Chapter. (1995). *Safe return survey evaluation report.* St. Louis, MO: Author.

Alzheimer's Disease and Related Disorders Association. (1990). *Fact sheets* [Brochure]. Chicago, IL: Author.

Alzheimer's Disease and Related Disorders Association. (1990). *Alzheimer's disease statistics* [Brochure]. Chicago, IL: Author.

Alzheimer's Disease and Related Disorders Association. (Winter, 1995). Home alone with Alzheimer's. *Alzheimer's Association National Newsletter, 15*(4), 5–7.

Alzheimer's Disease and Related Disorders Association. (1996). *Alzheimer's Association Safe Return: For their safety, for your peace of mind* [Brochure]. Chicago, IL: Author.

Alzheimer's Disease and Related Disorders Association. (1997). Products and resources: A listing of items to assist Alzheimer's caregivers. *VII. Security Products* [On-line]. Available: http://www.alz.org.

Antonangeli, J. (1996). *Of two minds: A guide to the care of people with the dual diagnosis of Alzheimer's disease and mental retardation.* Cambridge, MA: Alzheimer's Association, Massachusetts Chapter.

Arno, S., & Frank, D. I. (1994). A group for "wandering" institutionalized clients with primary degenerative dementia. *Perspectives in Psychiatric Care, 30*(3), 13–16.

Assisted living for the aged and frail: Innovations in design, management, and financing. V. Regnier, J. Hamilton, and S. Tatabe (Columbia University Press, 1995). Available at 1-800-944-UNIV.

Associated Press. (1999). *Doctors will advise DMVs of patients who are risky drivers.* San Diego, CA: Author.

Associated Press. (1997). Psychiatrists recommend Alzheimer's patients forgo driving. Washington, DC: Author.

Ballard, C. G., Mohan, R. C., Bannister, C., Handy, S., & Patel, A. (1991). Wandering in dementia sufferers. *International Journal of Geriatric Psychiatry, 6*(8), 611–614.

Bandura, A. (1973). *Social learning theory.* Englewood Cliffs, NJ: Prentice Hall.

Becker, M. H., & Maiman, L. A. (1975). Sociobehavioral determinants of compliance with health and medical care recommendations. *Medical Care, 13,* 10–24.

Berg, L., & Morris, J. C. (1994). Diagnosis. In R. D. Terry, R. Katzman, & K. Bick (Eds.), *Alzheimer's Disease* (pp. 9–25). New York: Raven Press, Ltd.

Berky, P. S. (1991). Alzheimer's by moonlight. *Geriatric Nursing, 12*(6), 292–293.

Bonifazi, W. Out for a walk. *Contemporary Long-Term Care, 23*, 40–46.

Bonner, A. P., & Cousins, S. (1996). Exercise and Alzheimer's disease: Benefits and barriers. *Activities, Adaptations and Aging, 20*(4), 21–35.

Boston Police Department. (1992). *Boston police rules and procedures manual*, Rule 17: Lost children and missing persons (amended by Special Order 92-2, Dec. 30). Boston, MA: Author.

Brawley, E. (1997). Wandering guidelines. In *Designing for Alzheimer's disease.* New York, NY: John Wiley & Sons.

Breitner, J. C. S., Wyse, B. W., Anthony, J. C., Welsh-Bohmer, K. A., & Steffens, D. C. (1999). APOE-e4 count predicts age when prevalence of AD increases, then declines. *Neurology, 53*(2), 321–330.

Brenner, D. E., et al. (1994). Postmenopausal estrogen replacement therapy and the risk of Alzheimer's disease: A population-based case-control study. *American Journal of Epidemiology,* (Aug. 1), 140(3), 262–267.

Bruck, L. (1995). Wanderer departure systems: High-tech, low-worry. *Nursing Homes, 44*(2), 32–35.

Burns, A., Jacoby, R., & Levy, R. (1990). Psychiatric phenomena in Alzheimer's disease. *British Journal of Psychiatry, 157,* 86–94.

Burnside, I. (1981). Touching is talking. *American Journal of Nursing, 73,* 2060–2063.

Butler, J. P., & Barnett, C. A. (1991). Window of wandering. *Geriatric Nursing, 12,* 226–227.

Caldwell, M. D. (1995). *Gone without a trace.* Forest Knolls, CA: Elder Books.

Calkins, M. P. (1988). Behavior changes: Wandering. In *Design for dementia: Planning environments for the elderly and confused.* Owings Mills, MD: National Health Publishing Co.

Calkins, M. P., & Namazi, K. H. (1991). Caregivers' perceptions of the effectiveness of home modifications for community living adults with dementia. *The American Journal of Alzheimer's Care and Related Disorders & Research, 6*(1), 25–29.

Cantor, M. (1980). The informal support system, its relevance in the lives of the elderly. In E. Borgatta & N. McCloskey (Eds.), *Aging and society* (pp. 131–144). Beverly Hills: Sage.

Chaftez, P. K. (1991). Structuring environments for dementia patients. In M. F. Weiner (Ed.), *The dementias: Diagnosis and management.* Washington, DC: American Psychiatric Press.

Chenoweth, B., & Spencer, B. (1986). Dementia: The experience of family caregivers. *The Gerontologist, 26*(3), 267–272.

Cobb, R. W., & Coughlin, J. F. (1997). Regulating older drivers: How are the states coping? *Journal of Aging & Social Policy, 9*(4), 71–87.

Cohen, U., & Day, K. (1993). Opportunities for meaningful wandering. In *Contemporary environments for people with dementia.* Baltimore, MD: Johns Hopkins University Press.

Cohen-Mansfield, J., Werner, P., Marx, M., & Freedman, L. (1991). Two studies of pacing in the nursing home. *Journal of Gerontology: Medical Sciences, 46*(3), M77–M83.

Cohen-Mansfield, J. W., Culpepper, W. J., Wolfson, M., & Bickel, E. (1997). Assessment of ambulatory behavior in nursing home residents who pace or wander: A comparison of four commercially available devices. *Dementia and Geriatric Cognitive Disorders, 8*(6), 359–365.

Cohen-Mansfield, J., & Werner, P. (1995). Environmental influences on agitation: An integrative summary of an observational study. *The American Journal of Alzheimer's Care and Related Disorders and Research, 10*(1), 32–39.

Collopy, B. J. (1995). Safe and unsound. *Contemporary Long-Term Care, 18*(8), 44–48.

Coltharp, W., Richie, M. F., & Kaas, M. J. (1996). Wandering. *Journal of Gerontological Nursing, 22,* 5–11.

Connell, B. R., & Sanford, J. A. (1994). Evaluation of interventions to prevent elopement among nursing home patients. *Rehabilitation R&D Progress Reports, 30–31,* 93–94.

Coombs, F. (1994). Engineering technology in rehabilitation of older adults. *Experimental Aging Research, 20,* 201–209.

Coombs, F., & Connell, B. R. (1994). A knowledge-based system for selecting elopement control devices. *Rehabilitation R&D Progress Reports, 30–31,* 91–92.

Coons, D. H. (1988). Wandering. *The American Journal of Alzheimer's Care and Related Disorders and Research, 3,* 31–36.

Cooper, J. K., Mungas, D., & Weiler, P. G. (1990). Relation of cognitive status and abnormal behaviors in Alzheimer's disease. *Journal of the American Geriatrics Society, 38,* 867–870.

Coulton, C. J. (1978). Factors related to preventive health behavior. *Social Work in Health Care, 3*(3), 297–310.

Crosby, L. J., Wyles, C. L., Verran, J. A., & Tynan, C. M. (1993). Taxonomy of evening and nighttime behavior patterns of persons with Alzheimer's disease. *The American Journal of Alzheimer's Care and Related Disorders and Research, 8*(2), 7–15.

Davidhizar, R., & Cosgray, R. (1990). Helping the wanderer. *Geriatric Nursing, 11*(6), 280–281.

Davidson, S. (1992). *The locator system for wandering individuals.* Houston, TX: NASA.

Davis, C. (1996). Making the most of wander-control technology. *Nursing Homes and Long-Term Care Management, 45*(2), 34–35.

Davis, L. (1991). Aiding the Alzheimer's dementia patient to live in safety and security. *Caring, 10,* 36–42.

Davis, R. (1989). *My journey into Alzheimer's disease: A story of hope.* Wheaton, IL: Tyndale Press.

Dawson, P., & Reid, D. W. (1987). Behavioral dimensions of patients at risk of wandering. *The Gerontologist, 27*(1), 104–107.

Day, N., Musallam, K., & Wells, M. (1999). Observed behaviors of patients with probable Alzheimer's disease who are hospitalized for diagnostic tests. *Journal of Gerontological Nursing, 25*(11), 35–39.

Day, K., Carreon, D., & Stump, C. (2000). The therapeutic design of environments for people with dementia: A review of the empirical research. *Gerontologist, 40,* 397–416.

Devor, M., Wang, A., Renvall, M., Feigal, D., & Ramsdell, J. (1994). Compliance with social and safety recommendations in an outpatient comprehensive geriatric assessment program. *Journal of Gerontology, 49*(104), M168–M173.

Dickinson, J. I., McLain-Kark, J., & Marshall-Baker, A. (1995). The effects of visual barriers on exiting behavior in a dementia care unit. *The Gerontologist, 35*(1), 127–130.

Dickinson, J. I., & McLain-Kark, J. (1998). Wandering behavior and attempted exits among residents diagnosed with dementia-related illnesses: A qualitative approach. *Journal of Women and Aging, 10,* 23–34.

DriveWise. (2001). *DriveWise: A Driving Fitness Evaluation Program.* Beth Israel Deaconess Medical Center, Boston, MA. Available: http://www.bidmc.caregroup.org/DriveWise.asp

Duffy, C. J., Tetewsky, S. J., & O'Brien, H. (2000). Cortical motion blindness in visuospatial AD. *Neurobiology of Aging, 21*(6), 867–870.

Epstein, B. D. (1994). Wandering and liability revisited. *Provider,* pp. 41–43.

Evans, D., Funkenstein, H., Albert, M., Scherr, P., Cook, N., Chown, M., Herbert, L., Hennekens, C., & Taylor, J. (1989). Prevalence of Alzheimer's disease in a community population of older persons. *Journal of the American Medical Association, 262,* 2551–2556.

Evans, D. A., Scherr, P. A., & Cook, N. R. (1990). Estimated prevalence of Alzheimer's disease in the United States. *Millbank Memorial Fund Quarterly, 68,* 267–289.

Ferris, S. H., Steinberg, G., Shulman, E., Kahn, R., & Reisberg, B. (1987). Institutionalization of Alzheimer's disease patients: Reducing precipitating factors through family counseling. *Home Health Services Quarterly, 8,* 23–51.

Finkel, S. I. (1993). Behavioral problems in dementia patients. *Geriatric Consultant, 10*(4), 27–29.

Flaherty, G., & Raia, P. (1994). Beyond risk: Protection and Alzheimer's disease. *Journal of Elder Abuse and Neglect, 6,* 75–93.

Flaherty, G., & Scheft, J. (1995). *Law enforcement, Alzheimer's disease & the lost elder.* Cambridge, MA: Alzheimer's Association, Massachusetts Chapter.

Fleiss, J. L., Williams, J. B., & Dubro, A. F. (1986). Logistic regression of psychiatric data. *Journal of Psychiatric Research, 20,* 145–209.

Foltz-Gray, D. (1997). One step at a time. *Contemporary Long-Term Care, 20,* 54–59.

Freedman, M., & Freedman, D. (1996). Should Alzheimer's disease patients be allowed to drive? A medical, legal, and ethical dilemma. *Journal of the American Geriatrics Society, 44,* 876–877.

Fried, T. R., Rosenberg, R., & Lipsitz, L. A. (1995). Older community-dwelling adults' attitudes toward and practices of health promotion and advance planning activities. *Journal of the American Geriatrics Society, 43,* 645–669.

Friedman, R., & Tappan, R. M. (1991). The effect of planned walking on communication in Alzheimer's disease. *Journal of the American Geriatrics Society, 39*(7), 650–654.

Gaffney, J. (1986). Toward a less restrictive environment. *Geriatric Nursing, 7,* 94–96.

Garling, A., & Garling, T. (1993). Mothers' supervision and perception of young children's risk of unintentional injury in the home. *Journal of Pediatric Psychology, 18*(1), 105–114.

Gillespie, N. D., & McMurdok, M. E. (1999). A survey of attitudes and knowledge of geriatricians to driving in elderly patients. *Age and Ageing, 28,* 53–57.

Gilley, D. W., Wilson, R. S., Beckett, L. A., & Evans, D. A. (1997). Psychotic symptoms and physically aggressive behavior in Alzheimer's disease. *Journal of the American Geriatric Society, 45*(9), 1074–1079.

Gillins, L. (1990). Yielding to age: When the elderly can no longer drive. *Journal of Gerontological Nursing, 16*(11), 12–17.

Gitlin, L. N., & Corcoran, M. A. (1996). Managing dementia at home: The role of home environmental modifications. *Topics in Geriatric Rehabilitation, 12*(2), 28–39.

Gofin, R., Palti, H., & Adler, B. (1990). The use of car restraints by newborns and mothers: Knowledge, attitudes, and practices. *Israel Journal of Medical Sciences, 26*(5), 261–265.

Gofin, R., Israeli, I., & Palti, H. (1991). The incidence of childhood and adolescent injuries and the outcome: A population-based study. *Israel Journal of Medical Sciences, 27*(10), 566–571.

Goldsmith, S. M., Hoeffer, B., & Rader, J. (1995). Problematic wandering behavior in the cognitively impaired elderly. *Journal of Psychosocial Nursing and Mental Health Services, 33*(2), 6–12.

Groene, R. (1993). Effectiveness of music therapy: 1:1 intervention with individuals having senile dementia of the Alzheimer's type. *Journal of Music Therapy, 30,* 138–157.

Grusec, J. E. (1992). Social learning theory and developmental psychology: The legacies of Robert Sears and Albert Bandura. *Developmental Psychology, 28*(5), 776–786.

Haley, W. E., & Coleton, M. L. (1992). Alzheimer's disease: Special issues in elder abuse and neglect. *Journal of Elder Abuse and Neglect, 4*(4), 71–85.

Hall, G. R., Buckwalter, K. C., Stolley, J. M., Gerdner, L. A., Garand, L., Ridgeway, S., & Crump, S. (1995). Standardized care plan: Managing Alzheimer's patients at home. *Journal of Gerontological Nursing, 21*, 37–47.

Hall, G. R. (1999). Outside the box: Restraint alternatives that work in acute care. Handout. Mayo Clinic, Scottsdale, AZ.

Health Care Financing Administration. (1989). Medicare and Medicaid: Requirements for long-term care facilities. *Federal Register,* 54, 5316–5336.

Heard, K., & Watson, T. S. (1999). Reducing wandering by persons with dementia using differential reinforcement. *Journal of Applied Behavior Analysis, 32,* 381–384.

Hearthstone Alzheimer Care. (1998). *SCU self-assessment workbook.* Lexington, MA: Author.

Heim, K. M. (1986). Wandering behavior. *Journal of Gerontological Nursing, 12*(11), 4–7.

Hiatt, L. G. (1985). *Interventions and people who wander: Contradictions in practice.* Paper presented at the 38th scientific meeting of the Gerontological Society of America, New Orleans, LA.

Hill, K. (1991). Predicting the behavior of lost persons. NASAR Conference Proceeding. NASAR: Fairfax, VA.

Hinrichsen, G. A., & Ramirez, M. (1992). Black and white dementia caregivers: A comparison of their adaptation, adjustment, and service utilization. *The Gerontologist, 32*(3), 375–381.

Hirschfeld, M. J. (1985). Ethics and care for the elderly. *International Journal of Nursing Studies, 22*(4), 319–328.

Hoffman, S. B., & Platt, C. A. (1990). Wandering. In S. B. Hoffman & C. A. Platt, *Comforting the confused: Strategies for managing dementia.* New York: Springer Publishing.

Hoffman, S. B., Platt, C. A., & Barry, K. E. (1987). Managing the difficult dementia patient: The impact on untrained nursing home staff. *American Journal of Alzheimer's Care and Related Disorders Research, 2*(4), 26–31.

Holden, G. (1991). The relationship of self-efficacy appraisals to subsequent health related outcomes: A meta-analysis. *Social Work in Health Care, 16*(1), 53–93.

Holmberg, S. K. (1997). Walking program for wanderers: Volunteer training and development of an evening walker's group. *Geriatric Nursing, 18*, 160–165.

Hofland, B. F. (1994). When capacity fades and autonomy is constricted: A client-centered approach to residential care. *Generations, 18*(4), 31–35.

Hope, R. A., & Fairburn, C. G. (1990). The nature of wandering in dementia: A community-based study. *International Journal of Geriatric Psychiatry, 5*, 239–245.

Hope, T., Tilling, K., & Fairburn, C. G. (1994). The structure of wandering in dementia. *International Journal of Geriatric Psychiatry, 9*, 149–155.

Horowitz, A. (1985). Family caregiving to the frail elderly. In M. P. Lawton & G. Maddox (Eds.), *Annual Review of Gerontology and Geriatrics, 5*, 194–246. New York: Springer Publishing.

Horowitz, A., Silverstone, B. A., & Reinhardt, J. P. (1991). A conceptual and empirical exploration of personal autonomy issues within family caregiving relationships. *The Gerontologist, 31*(1), 23–32.

Hunt, L., Morris, J. C., Edwards, D., & Wilson, B. S. (1993). Driving performance in persons with mild senile dementia of the Alzheimer type. *Journal of the American Geriatrics Society, 41,* 747–752.

Hussian, R. A. (1982–83). Stimulus control in the modification of problematic behavior in elderly institutionalized patients. *International Journal of Behavior Geriatrics, 1,* 33–42.

Hussian, R. A., & Brown, D. C. (1987). Use of two-dimensional grid to limit hazardous ambulation in demented patients. *Journal of Gerontology, 42,* 558–560.

I.D.E.A.S., Inc., 1600 Rydalmount Rad, Cleveland Heights, OH 44118-1352; 216-791-4648 (phone); 216-791-4843 (fax); *IDEASmpc@aol.com* (email address). For information on Remodel, a National Institute on Aging-funded project to develop a more efficient method of creating more supportive physical environments for long-term care residents with dementia. Can also order Design for Dementia (National Health Publishing, 1988), a design guide for dementia care units by Margaret P. Calkins.

Johansson, K., Bogdanovic, N., Kalimo, H., Winblad, B., & Viitanen, M. (1997). High incidence of Alzheimer pathology and apolipoprotein E e4-allele found in older drivers who died in automobile crashes. *Lancet, 349,* 1143–1144.

Johansson, K., Bronge, L., Lundberg, C., Persson, A., Seideman, M., & Viitanen, M. (1996). Can a physician recognize an older driver with increased crash risk potential? *Journal of the American Geriatrics Society, 44,* 1198–1204.

Kapp, M. B. (1995). Legal and ethical issues in home-based care. *Journal of Gerontological Social Work, 24*(3/4), 31–45.

Kapust, L. R., & Weintraub, S. (1992). To drive or not to drive: Preliminary results from road testing of patients with dementia. *Journal of Geriatric Psychiatry and Neurology, 5,* 128–131.

Karcher, K. (1993). Is your risk management program designed to deal with Alzheimer's disease? *Nursing Homes, 42*, 34–36.

Kasper, J., & Shore, A. D. (1994). Cognitive impairment and problem behaviors as risk factors for institutionalization. *Journal of Applied Gerontology, 13*(4), 371–385.

Kelly, T. B. (1994). Paternalism and the marginally competent: An ethical dilemma, no easy answers. *Journal of Gerontological Social Work, 23*(1/2), 67–84.

Kennedy, D. B. (1993). Precautions for the physical security of the wandering patient. *Security Journal, 4*(4), 170–176.

Kindig, M. N., & Carnes, M. (1993). Behavioral changes: Wandering. In *Coping with Alzheimer's disease and other dementing illnesses.* San Diego, CA: Springer Publishing.

King, T., & Mallet, L. (1991). Brachial plexus palsy with the use of haloperidolanda geriatric chair. *The Annals of Pharmacotherapy, 25*(10), 1072–1073.

Klein, D. A., Steinberg, M., Galik, E., Steele, C., Sheppard, J., Warren, A., Rosenblatt, A., & Lyketsos, C. G. (1999). Wandering behaviour in community-residing persons with dementia. *International Journal of Geriatric Psychiatry, 14,* 272–279.

Koester, R. J. (1999). *Lost Alzheimer's Disease Search Management: The law enforcement guide to managing the initial response and investigation of the missing Alzheimer's disease subject.* (Instructor's manual). Charlottesville, VA: dbs Productions.

Koester, R. J. (2001). Alzheimer's disease and related disorders SAR research: Wandering overview (How big is the problem?). http://www.dbs-sar.com.

Koester, R. J., & Stooksbury, D. E. (1995). Behavioral profile of possible Alzheimer's disease patients in Virginia search and rescue incidents. *Wilderness and Environmental Medicine, 6*(1), 34–43.

Kosberg, J. I., & Cairl, R. E. (1992). Burden and competence in caregivers of Alzheimer's disease patients: Research and practice implications. *Journal of Gerontological Social Work, 18*(1/2), 85–96.

Kulash, D. (2000). *Safe mobility for a maturing society: A strategic plan and national agenda.* Chapter for inclusion in the Transportation Research Board proceedings from the International Conference, Transportation in an Aging Society: A Decade of Experience, November 1999.

Kunkenmueller, P. (1998). A caregiver's odyssey. *Alzheimer's Association, Massachusetts Chapter Newsletter, 16*(1–2), 4–5.

Lach, H. W., Reed, A. T., Smith, L. J., & Carr, D. B. (1995). Alzheimer's disease: Assessing safety problems in the home. *Geriatric Nursing, 16*(4), 160–164.

Lai, F. (1992). Clinical pathological features of Alzheimer's disease in Down syndrome. *Down Syndrome and Alzheimer's Disease* (15–34). New York: Wiley-Liss.

Lawton, M. P., Fulcomer, M., & Kleban, M. (1984). Architecture for the mentally impaired elderly. *Environment and Behavior, 16*(6), 730–757.

LeMaire, D., & Lacy, R. (1994). Patience is a virtue. *Caring, 13*(8), 60–62.

LePore, P. R. (2000). *When you are concerned: A handbook for families, friends and caregivers worried about the safety of an aging driver* (pp. 1–53). Albany: New York State Office for the Aging.

Lewin, K. (1951). *Field theory in social science.* New York: Harper.

Lipscomb, H. S. (1988). Dementia: Helping families cope. *Caring, 7*(7), 28–29.

Logsdon, R., Teri, L., McCurry, S. M., Gibbons, L. E., Kukull, W. A., & Larson, E. B. (1998). Wandering: A significant problem among community-residing individuals with Alzheimer's disease. *Journal of Gerontology, 53B*(5), P294–P299.

Lombardo, N. E. (1997). Routes of hope: Report on the 7th Matthew and Marcia Simons annual research lecture. *Alzheimer's Association, Massachusetts Chapter Newsletter, 15*(4), 3.

Lucas-Blaustein, M. J., Filipp, L., Dungan, C., & Tune, L. (1988). Driving in patients with dementia. *Journal of the American Geriatrics Society, 36*(12), 1087–1091.

Lucero, M., Hutchinson, S., Leger-Krall, S., & Wilson, H. S. (1993). Wandering in Alzheimer's dementia patients. *Clinical Nursing Research, 2*(2), 160–175.

Mace, N. L., & Rabins, P. V. (1991). Problems of behavior: Wandering. In *The 36-hour day.* Baltimore, MD: Johns Hopkins University Press.

Madson, J. (1991). The study of wandering in persons with senile dementia. *The American Journal of Alzheimer's Care and Related Disorders and Research, 6,* 21–24.

Martin, B. (1993). New technology makes wandering safer: Departure alert monitors are broadening in scope and accuracy. *Nursing Homes, 42*(4), 11–14.

Martino-Saltzman, D., Blasch, B. B., Morris, R. D., & McNeal, L. W. (1991). Travel behavior of nursing home residents perceived as wanderers and nonwanderers. *The Gerontologist, 31*(5), 666–672.

Matteson, M. A., Linton, A., & Byers, V. (1993). Vision and hearing screening in cognitively impaired older adults. *Geriatric Nursing, 14*, 294–297.

Mayer, R., & Darby, S. J. (1991). Does a mirror deter wandering in demented older people? *International Journal of Geriatric Psychiatry, 6*, 607–609.

McCarten, J. R., Kovera, C., Maddox, M. K., & Cleary, J. P. (1995). Triazolam in Alzheimer's disease: Pilot study on sleep and memory effects. *Pharmacology, Biochemistry and Behavior, 52*(2), 447.

McConnell, E. A. (1998). Managing patient falls and wandering. *Nursing Management, 29*(8), 75.

McGlynn, S. M., & Schacter, D. L. (1989). Unawareness of deficits in neuropsychological syndromes. *Journal of Clinical Experimental Neuropsychology, 11,* 143–205.

McShane, R., Hope, T., & Wilkinson, J. (1994). Tracking patients who wander: Ethics and technology. *The Lancet, 343,* 1274.

McShane, R., Gedling, K., Kenward, B., Kenward, R., Hope, T., & Jacoby, R. (1998). The feasibility of electronic tracking devices in dementia: A telephone survey and case series. *International Journal of Geriatric Psychiatry, 13*(8), 556–563.

Mellilo, K. D., & Futrell, M. (1998). Wandering and technology devices: Helping ensure the safety of confused older adults. *Journal of Gerontological Nursing, 24*(8), 32–38.

Mendez, M. F., Martin, R. J., Smyth, K. A., & Whitehouse, P. J. (1990). Psychiatric symptoms associated with Alzheimer's disease. *Journal of Neuropsychiatry, 2,* 28–33.

Miles, S. (1996). A case of death by physical restraint: New lessons from a photograph. *Journal of the American Geriatrics Society, 44*, 291–292.

Miller, D. J., & Morley, J. E. (1993). Attitudes of physicians toward elderly drivers and driving policy. *Journal of the American Geriatrics Society, 40,* 722–724.

Mittelman, M. S., Ferris, S. H., Steinberg, G., Shulman, E., Mackell, J. A., Ambinder, A., & Cohen, J. (1996). An intervention that delays institutionalization of Alzheimer's disease patients: Treatment of spouse-caregivers. *The Gerontologist, 33*(6), 730–740.

Monsour, N., & Robb, S. S. (1982). Wandering behavior in old age: A psychosocial study. *Social Work, 27,* 411–416.

Moretz, C., Dommel, A., & Deluca, K. (1995). Untied: A safe alternative to restraints. *Nursing, 4*(2), 128–132.

Morgan, D. G., & Stewart, N. J. (1999). The physical environment of special care units: Needs of residents with dementia from the perspective of staff and caregivers. *Qualitative Health Research, 9,* 105–118.

Morishita, L. (1990). Wandering behavior. In J. L. Cummings & B. L. Miller (Eds.), *Alzheimer's disease: Treatment and long-term care management.* New York: Marcel Dekker.

Morse, J. M., Tylko, S. J., & Dixon, H. A. (1987). Characteristics of the fall-prone patient. *The Gerontologist, 27,* 516–523.

Moss, M. B., & Albert, M. S. (1988). Alzheimer's disease and other dementing disorders. In M. S. Albert & M. B. Moss (Eds.), *Geriatric neuropsychology* (pp. 145–178). New York: The Guilford Press.

Myers, D. L. (1996). Remedies beyond counting sheep. *Provider, 22*(2), 62–64.

Namazi, K. H., & Johnson, B. D. (1992). Pertinent autonomy for residents with dementias: Modification of the physical environment to enhance independence. *American Journal of Alzheimer's Care and Related Disorders Research, 7,* 16–21.

Namazi, K. H., Rosner, T. T., & Calkins, M. P. (1989). Visual barriers to prevent ambulatory Alzheimer's patients from exiting through an emergency door. *The Gerontologist, 29,* 699–702.

Nasr, S., Tuck, J., & Osterweil, D. (1997). Nonpharmacologic management of wandering behavior in the nursing home: A consensus approach. *Annals of Long-Term Care, 5*(12), 401–411.

Negley, E. N., Molla, P. M., & Obenchain, J. (1990). No exit: The effects of an electronic security system on confused patients. *Journal of Gerontological Nursing, 16*(8), 21–25.

North Carolina Department of Health and Human Services Division on Aging. (March, 2000). *Acute hospitalization & Alzheimer's disease: A special kind of care.* Raleigh, NC: North Carolina Health and Human Services.

Noyes, L. E., & Silva, M. C. (1993). The ethics of locked special care units for persons with Alzheimer's disease. *The American Journal of Alzheimer's Care and Related Disorders & Research, 9,* 12–15.

O'Connor, M., & Kapust, L. (March 27, 2001). E-mail communication.

Ohta, R., & Ohta, B. (1990, November). *Factors affecting the acceptance and use of home adaptation by the elderly.* Paper presented at the meeting of the Gerontological Society of America, Boston, MA.

Ory, M. G., & Cox, D. M. (1994). Forging ahead: Linking health and behavior to improve quality of life in older people. *Social Indicators Research, 33,* 89–120.

Petro, J. A., Belger, D., Salzberg, C. A., & Salisbury, R. E. (1989). Burn accidents and the elderly: What is happening and how to prevent it. *Geriatrics, 44,* 26–48.

Pollack, C. P., & Perlick, D. (1987). Sleep problems and institutionalization of older persons. *Sleep Research, 16,* 407.

Pynoos, J., & Ohta, R. J. (1991). In-home interventions for persons with Alzheimer's disease and their caregivers. *Physical & Occupational Therapy in Geriatrics, 9*(3–4), 83–92.

Pynoos, J., Cohen, E., & Lucas, C. (1989). Environmental coping strategies for Alzheimer's caregivers. *The American Journal of Alzheimer's Care and Related Disorders & Research, 4,* 4–8.

Rabins, P. V., Mace, N. L., & Lucas, M. (1982). The impact of dementia on the family. *Journal of the American Medical Association, 248,* 333–335.

Radebaugh, T. S., Buckholtz, N., & Khachaturian, Z. (Eds.). (1996). Behavioral approaches to the treatment of Alzheimer's disease: Research strategies. *International Psychogeriatrics, 8*(1), 7–144.

Rader, J., Doan, J., & Schwab, M. (1985). How to decrease wandering, a form of agenda behavior. *Geriatric Nursing, 6*(4), 196–199.

Raia, P. A. (1994). Helping patients and families to take control. *Psychiatric Annals, 24*(4), 192.

Raia, P., & Koenig-Coste, J. (1996). Habilitation therapy: Realigning the planets. *Alzheimer's Association, Massachusetts Chapter Newsletter, 14*(2), 3–14.

Raschko, R. (1991). *Living alone with Alzheimer's disease: A social policy time-bomb.* (Monograph).

Reed, A. T., Lach, H. W., Smith, L., & Birge, S. J. (1990). Alzheimer's disease and the need for supervision. *The American Journal of Alzheimer's Care and Related Disorders & Research, 5*(5), 29–34.

Reiman, E. M. (1996). Preclinical evidence of Alzheimer's disease in persons homozygous for the e4 allele for apolipoprotein E. *The New England Journal of Medicine, 334*(12), 752–758.

Reuben, D. B., Silliman, R. A., & Traines, M. (1988). The aging driver. *Journal of the American Geriatrics Society, 36*, 1135–1142.

Richter, J. M., Roberto, K. A., & Bottenberg, D. J. (1995). Communicating with persons with Alzheimer's disease: Experiences of family and formal caregivers. *Archives of Psychiatric Nursing, 9*(5), 279–285.

Riekse, R. J., & Holstege, H. (1996). *Growing older in America.* New York: McGraw-Hill.

Roberto, K. (1994). Ethical challenges facing family caregivers of persons with Alzheimer's disease. *Activities, Adaptation and Aging, 18*(3/4), 49–61.

Roberts, B. L., & Algase, D. L. (1988). Victims of Alzheimer's disease and the environment. *The Nursing Clinics of North America, 23*(1), 83–93.

Roberts, C. (1996). The management of wandering in older people with dementia. *Journal of Psychiatric and Mental Health Nursing, 3*(2), 138–139.

Robinson, A., Spencer, B., & White, L. (1989). Understanding difficult behaviors: Some practical suggestions for coping with Alzheimer's disease and related illnesses. Ypsilanti, MI: Eastern Michigan University.

Rodriguez, J. (1993). Resident falls and elopement. *Nursing Homes, 42,* 16–17.

Rosa-Brady, J., & Dunne, T. (Fall/Winter 1999). Visual disorders and Alzheimer's: A closer look at a common problem. *Alzheimer's Association, Massachusetts Chapter Newsletter, 17*(3).

Rosen, J., & Zubenko, G. S. (1991). Emergence of psychosis and depression in the longitudinal evaluation of Alzheimer's disease. *Biological Psychiatry, 29*(3), 224.

Roses, A. D. (1995). Apolipoprotein E genotyping in the differential diagnosis, not prediction, of Alzheimer's disease. *Annals of Neurology, 38*(1), 6–14.

Ross, G. W., Petrovitch, H., & White, L. R. (1996–1997). Update on dementia. *Generations, 20*(4), 22–27.

Rosswurm, M. A., Zimmerman, S. L., Schwartz-Fulton, J., & Norman, G. A. (1986). Can we manage wandering behavior? *Journal of Long Term Care Administration, 14*, 58.

Rowe, M. A., & Glover, J. C. (2001). Cognitively impaired individuals who become lost in the community: A descriptive study of safe return discoveries. *American Journal of Alzheimer's Disease and Other Dementias, Nov/Dec*, 1–9.

Russell, K. M., & Champion, V. L. (1996). Health beliefs and social influence in home safety practices of mothers with preschool children. *Image—The Journal of Nursing Scholarship, 28*(1), 59–64.

Ryan, J. P., McGowan, J., McCaffrey, N., Ryan, T., Zandi, T., & Brannigan, G. G. (1995). Graphomotor perserveration and wandering in Alzheimer's disease. *Journal of Geriatric Psychiatry and Neurology, 8,* 209–212.

Sacks, O. (1985). *The man who mistook his wife for a hat and other clinical tales.* New York: Summit Books.

Salmons, T. (1999). *Wandering, getting lost, and Alzheimer's disease: Influences on precautions taken and levels of supervision provided by caregivers.* Unpublished dissertation, University of Massachusetts, Boston, MA.

Sanford, J. (1975). Tolerance of disability in elderly dependents by supporters at home: Its significance for hospital practice. *British Medical Journal, 3,* 471–473.

Selkoe, D. J. (1992). New hope and insight into what causes Alzheimer's disease: The 1st Matthew and Marcia Simons annual research lecture. *Alzheimer's Association, Massachusetts Chapter Newsletter, 10*(1–2), 4.

Shedd, P. P., Kobokovich, L. J., & Slattery, M. J. (1995). Confused patients in the acute care setting: Prevalence, interventions, and outcomes. *Journal of Gerontological Nursing, 21*(4), 5–12.

Schulz, R., O'Brien, A. T., Bookwala, J., & Fleissner, K. (1995). Psychiatric and physical morbidity effects of dementia caregiving: Prevalence, correlates, and causes. *The Gerontologist, 35*(6), 771–791.

Schweitzer, S. O., Atchison, K. A., Lubben, J. E., Mayer-Oakes, S. A., De Jong, F. J., & Matthias, R. E. (1994). Health promotion and disease prevention for older adults: Opportunity for change or preaching to the converted? *American Journal of Preventive Medicine, 10*(4), 223–229.

Shanas, E. (1979). Social myth as hypothesis: The case of the family relations of old people. *The Gerontologist, 19,* 3–9.

Shemon, K., & Christensen, R. (1991). Automobile driving and Alzheimer's disease. *The American Journal of Alzheimer's Care and Related Disorders & Research, 6*(5), 3–8.

Shneider, M. A. (1998). What to do for wandering. *Caring, 17*(7), 40–41.

Shooper, S. S. (1991). Caregivers of Alzheimer's disease patients: A review of the literature. *Journal of Gerontological Social Work, 18*(1–2), 19–37.

Silverstein, N. M. (1984). Informing the elderly about public services: The relationship between sources of knowledge and service utilization. *The Gerontologist, 24*(1), 37–40.

Silverstein, N. M., & Salmons, T. (1996). *He comes back eventually: Wandering behavior in community-residing persons with Alzheimer's disease registered in Safe Return.* Boston: University of Massachusetts-Boston, Gerontology Institute.

Silverstein, N. M., & Hyde, J. (1997). The importance of a consumer perspective in home adaptation of Alzheimer's households. In S. Lanspery & J. Hyde (Eds.), *Staying Put: Adapting the Places Instead of the People* (pp. 91–111). Amityville, NY: Baywood Publishing Company.

Silverstein, N. M., Hyde, J., & Ohta, R. (1993). Home adaptation for Alzheimer's households: Factors related to implementation and outcomes of recommendations. *Technology and Disability, 2*(4), 58–68.

Silverstein, N. M., Bruner-Canhoto, L., Goldberg, K., Greenan, K., Hogan, P., Kabba, U., Lojek, M., MacDonald, M., MacNeill, J., Pohotsky, D., Toomey, J., & Weistrop, J. (2000). *How "dementia-friendly" are acute care hospital stays in Massachusetts.* Poster presented at the Alzheimer's Association, Massachusetts Chapter, Annual Multidisciplinary Conference for Professionals, A Map Through the Maze, Marlboro, MA.

Silverstein, N. M., & Murtha, J. (2001). *Driving in Massachusetts: When to stop and who should decide?* Boston: University of Massachusetts Boston, Gerontology Institute.

Sims, R. V., Owsley, C., Allman, R. M., Ball, K., & Smoot, T. M. (1998). A preliminary assessment of the medical and functional factors associated with vehicle crashes by older adults. *Journal of the American Geriatrics Society, 46,* 556–561.

Small, G. W., Rabins, P. V., Barry, P. P., Buckholtz, N. S., DeKosky, S. T., Ferris, S. H., et al. (1997). Diagnosis and treatment of Alzheimer's disease and related disorders: Consensus statement of the American Association for Geriatric Psychiatry, the Alzheimer's Association, and the American Geriatrics Society. *Journal of the American Medical Society*, (Oct. 22/29), *278*(16), 1363–1371.

Snowdon, D., Kemper, S., Mortimer, J., Greiner, L., Wekstein, D., & Markesberg, W. (1996). Linguistic ability in early life and cognitive function and Alzheimer's disease in late life: Findings from the Nun study. *Journal of the American Medical Association, 275*(7), 528–532.

Snyder, L. H., Rupprecht, P., Pyrek, J., Brekhus, S., & Moss, T. (1978). Wandering. *The Gerontologist, 18,* 272–280.

Souren, L. E. M., Franssen, E. H., & Reisberg, B. (1995). Contractures and loss of function in patients with Alzheimer's disease. *Journal of the American Geratrics Society, 43*(6), 650–655.

Steele, C., Rovner, B., Chase, G. A., & Folstein, M. (1990). Psychiatric symptoms and nursing home placement of patients with Alzheimer's disease. *American Journal of Psychiatry, 147,* 1049–1051.

Stehman, J., Strachman, G., Glenner, G., & Neubaur, J. (1996). *Handbook of dementia care.* Baltimore, MD: Johns Hopkins University Press.

Stewart, J. T. (1995). Management of behavior problems in the demented patient. *American Family Physician, 52*(8), 2311–2320.

Stoppe, G., Sandholzer, H., Staedt, J., Winter, S., Kiefer, J., & Ruther, E. (1995). Sleep disturbances in the demented elderly: Treatment in ambulatory care. *Sleep, 18*(10), 844–848.

Stutts, J. C. (1998). Do older drivers with visual and cognitive impairments drive less? *Journal of the American Geriatrics Society, 46,* 854–861.

Sutor, B., Rummans, T. A., & Smith, G. E. (2001). Assessment and management of behavioral disturbances in nursing home patients with dementia. *Mayo Clin Proceedings, 76,* 540–550.

Tabachnick, B. F., & Fidell, L. S. (1989). *Using multivariate statistics* (2nd ed.). New York: Harper Collins.

Taft, L. B., Delaney, K., Seman, D., & Stansell, J. (1993). Dementia care: Creating a therapeutic milieu. *Journal of Gerontological Nursing, 19*(10), 30–33.

Tangalos, E. G. (1999). Transitioning the patient in and out of acute care. Workshop presentation, Boston Alzheimer's Symposium. October 16, 1999. Boston Museum of Science, Boston, MA.

Teri, L., Larson, E. B., & Reifler, B. V. (1988). Behavioral disturbance in dementia of the Alzheimer's type. *Journal of Applied Gerontology, 36,* 1–6.

Teri, L., Borson, S., Kiyak, A., & Yamagishi, M. (1989). Behavioral disturbance, cognitive dysfunction, and functional skill: Prevalence and relationship in Alzheimer's disease. *Journal of the American Geriatrics Society, 37*(2), 110–116.

Teri, L., Rabins, P., Whitehouse, P., Berg, L., Reisberg, B., Sunderland, T., Eichelman, B., & Phelps, C. (1992). Management of behavior disturbances in Alzheimer's disease: Current knowledge and future directions. *Alzheimer's Disease and Related Disorders, 6*(2), 77–88.

Tetewsky, S. J., & Duffy, C. J. (1999). Visual loss and getting lost in Alzheimer's disease. *Neurology, 52*(5), 958–964.

Thomas, D. W. (1997). Understanding the wandering patient: A continuity of personality perspective. *Journal of Gerontological Nursing, 23*(1), 16–24.

Thomas, D. W. (1995). Wandering: A proposed definition. *Journal of Gerontological Nursing, 21*(9), 35–41.

Tierney, M. C., Fisher, R. H., Lewis, A. J., et al. (1988). The NINCSDS-ADRDA work group criteria for the clinical diagnosis of probable Alzheimer's disease: A clinical pathologic study of 57 cases. *Neurology, 38,* 359–364.

U.S. Census Bureau. (12 February 1999). 1990 Census of Population and Housing, Summary Tape File 1 and Summary Tape File 3A, generated by Terri Salmons using 1990 Census Lookup, <http://venus.census.gov/cdrom/lookup>.

U.S. Congress, Office of Technology Assessment. (1990). *Confused minds, burdened families: Finding help for people with Alzheimer's & other dementias* (OTA-BA-403). Washington, DC: U.S. Government Printing Office.

U.S. Congress, Office of Technology Assessment. (1987). *Losing a million minds: Confronting the tragedy of Alzheimer's disease and other dementias* (OTA-BA-323). Washington, DC: U.S. Government Printing Office.

Vaughan, E., & Seifert, M. (1992). Variability in the framing of risk issues. *Journal of Social Issues, 48*(4), 119–135.

Virginia Department of Criminal Justice Services. (2000). Report to the House of Delegates Appropriations Committee and the Senate Finance Committee: Study on protecting individuals with Alzheimer's disease (October 2). Richmond, VA: Author.

Visser, H. (1983). Gait and balance in senile dementia of Alzheimer's type. *Age and Ageing, 12,* 296–301.

Wagner, J. S. (1996). Wandering and fall prevention: New solutions to a perennial problem. *Nursing, 26*(8), 24.

Watzke, J., & Smith, D. B. (1994). Concern for and knowledge of safety hazards among older people: Implications for research and prevention. *Experimental Aging Research, 20*(3), 177–188.

Weese, B. (1995). Fire and burn safety: Important issues for caregivers. *Caring Magazine, 14*(9), 40–42.

Werner, P., Cohen-Mansfield, J., Braun, J., & Marx, M. S. (1989). Physical restraints and agitation in nursing home residents. *Journal of the American Geriatrics Society, 37*(12), 1122–1126.

Wickersty, A. G. (1986). Wandering is number one behavioral problem, nursing home survey finds. *Nursing Home Security and Safety Management,* 1–3.

Wortel, E., De Geus, G. H., Kok, G., & Van Woerkum, C. (1994). Injury control in preschool children: A review of parental safety measures to prevent injuries on preschool children. *Health Education Research, 9*(2), 201–205.

Young, S. H., Muir-Nash, J., & Ninos, M. (1988). Managing nocturnal wandering behavior. *Journal of Gerontological Nursing, 14*(5), 6–12.

Zagami, J. M., Parl, S. A., Bussgang, J. J., & Mellilo, K. D. (1998). Providing universal location services using a wireless E911 location network. *IEEE Communications Magazine, 36*(4), 66–71.

Zeisel, J., Hyde, J., & Levkoff, S. (1994, March/April). Best practices: An environment-behavior model (E-B) for Alzheimer special care units. *The American Journal of Alzheimer's Care and Related Disorders & Research, 9*(2), 4–21.

Index